Supplements for Strength-Power Athletes

Supplements for Strength-Power Athletes

Jose Antonio, PhD, CSCS
Jeffrey R. Stout, PhD, CSCS*D

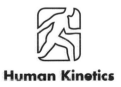

Human Kinetics

Library of Congress Cataloging-in-Publication Data

Antonio, Jose, PhD.
    Supplements for strength-power athletes / by Jose Antonio, Jeffrey R. Stout.
    p. cm.
Includes bibliographical references
    ISBN 0-7360-3772-1
    1. Dietary supplements. 2. Athletes--Nutrition. I. Stout, Jeffrey R. II. Title.

RM258.5.A5 A58 2002
613.2'088'796--dc21

                                    2002017329

ISBN: 0-7360-3772-1

Acquisitions Editor: Michael S. Barhke, PhD; **Developmental Editors:** D.K. Bihler and Myles Schrag; **Assistant Editor:** Lee Alexander; **Copyeditor:** Scott J. Weckerly; **Proofreader:** Sue Fetters; **Permission Manager:** Dalene Reeder; **Graphic Designer:** Nancy Rasmus; **Graphic Artist:** Dawn Sills; **Photo Manager:** Leslie A. Woodrum; **Cover Designer:** Keith Blomberg; **Photographer (cover):** Dick Young/Unicorn Stock Photos; **Photographer (interior):** Tom Roberts p. 4, 8, 29, 36, 40, 45, 52, 76, 83, 87, 90, 95; Terry Wild p. viii, 100; Leslie A. Woodrum p. 10.; **Art Manager:** Carl D. Johnson and Kelly R. Hendren; **Illustrator:** Craig Newsom; **Printer:** United Graphics

Printed in the United States of America   10 9 8 7 6 5 4 3 2 1

Human Kinetics
Web site: www.humankinetics.com

United States: Human Kinetics
P.O. Box 5076
Champaign, IL 61825-5076
800-747-4457
e-mail: humank@hkusa.com

Canada: Human Kinetics
475 Devonshire Road Unit 100
Windsor, ON N8Y 2L5
800-465-7301 (in Canada only)
e-mail: orders@hkcanada.com

Europe: Human Kinetics
107 Bradford Road
Stanningley
Leeds LS28 6AT, United Kingdom
+44 (0) 113 255 5665
e-mail: hk@hkeurope.com

Australia: Human Kinetics
57A Price Avenue
Lower Mitcham, South Australia 5062
08 8277 1555
e-mail: liahka@senet.com.au

New Zealand: Human Kinetics
P.O. Box 105-231, Auckland Central
09-523-3462
e-mail: hkp@ihug.co.nz

Contents

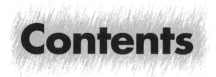

Part II Supplement Combinations

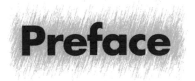

Preface

Sports nutrition and supplementation is a multibillion dollar industry that continues to expand. Because of this tremendous growth, there is a need for credible scientific information concerning the various ergogenic aids (i.e., a nutrient or supplement that enhances exercise or athletic performance) currently on the market. The popularity of magazines such as *Muscle and Fitness, Testosterone.net, Planet Muscle, Shape, Ironman, MuscleMag International, Muscle Media, Body International, Power,* and others demonstrate the high demand for information in the field of fitness. When you peruse these magazines, it is not uncommon to find articles written by those with little or no actual training in the scientific method. As a consumer, you are sometimes limited in where to get your information: From the clerk behind the counter of a health food store, a fitness writer with training in journalism, or perhaps an athlete who endorses a product (although one would be skeptical if he or she even consumed the product).

This book gives you an alternative, but what we present is certainly not written in stone. We realize that the area of sports supplementation is in constant flux. For instance, if you've ever spent time reading a scientific publication, often the concluding paragraph or sentence includes the clichéd phrase "more research is needed to determine if supplement x, y, and z . . ." Fill in the proverbial blanks. Of course more research is always needed; however, athletes and those who give advice to athletes (nutritionists, exercise physiologists, coaches) do not necessarily have the time to wait for scientists to come to a consensus on what works and what doesn't.

As an alternative, athletes can formulate a nutrition and supplementation plan using a mixture of science, trial and error, and just plain intuition. So for those of you who are science purists, you may find the idea of providing supplement advice (based on limited data or knowledge) a bit antithetical. But with limited data and time (the career of many professional athletes rarely spans more than a decade), it is critical that we

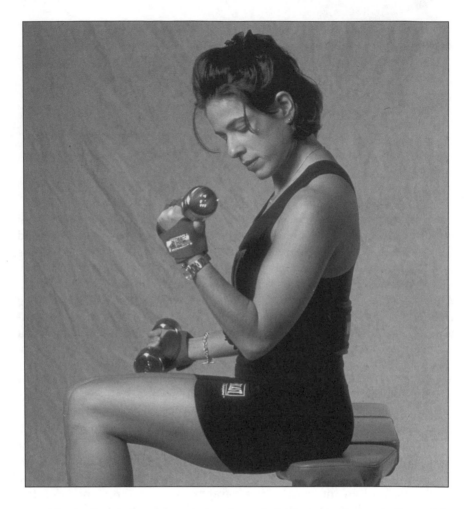

provide the best information to our knowledge on supplements that might improve performance. To hide behind the notion of "more research is needed"—and therefore not offer advice—would be nothing less than intellectual laziness.

Our book offers practical information in an easy-to-follow format. Athletes, coaches, trainers, and other allied health professionals will find this book informative and to-the-point. Two categories of supplements are discussed: single supplements and supplement combinations. Each supplement is listed alphabetically and is explained in five separate subheads.

- **What Is It?**

  In this section, each supplement is defined in chemical terms.

- **How Does It Work?**

  In this section, we present the theoretical basis for how this supplement may help a strength-power athlete.

- **The Evidence: Pro or Con?**

  In this section, we present the latest scientific studies that support or refute the efficacy of a particular supplement.

- **Guidelines for Use**

  In this section, we provide practical advice regarding the potential use of a supplement.

- **Precautions**

  In this section, we mention briefly the possible side effects that a supplement might have.

If you wish, you can skip any sections you find uninteresting and go straight to the bottom line—the "Guidelines for Use." (Of course, we hope you will find all of the information insightful.) You can choose to accept our recommendations, or you can choose not to accept them. Though we are trained as research scientists, we also value the trial-and-error information garnered by athletes. The scientific purist may cringe at the thought of using such anecdotal information, but it is often the case that the athletes who use supplements or combinations of supplements long before science can confirm or deny their benefits. For instance, strength-power athletes, particularly bodybuilders, have been consuming high-protein diets (more than twice the RDA) over the last 50 years, yet it has only been in the last 15 to 20 years that scientists have "confirmed" the need for extra protein. Therefore, it would be foolhardy to completely ignore the actual dietary practices of athletes. Besides, they're the ones who pay the price for choosing to use (or not use) a particular supplement. It is all too easy for scientists to state that dietary supplements are generally a waste of time and money, but the career of a scientist is not affected by whether they personally use or endorse a particular supplement. In the athletic field, it is quite different. If using a supplement confers even the smallest advantage, it may make the difference between winning and losing.

In addition, the question of whether supplement use is ethical or not is not as simple to address. Is taking creatine to enhance muscle strength and power ethical? If you eat a lot of meat, you get a lot of creatine, too. Is taking extra carbohydrates during an athletic event ethical? Clearly, carbohydrate supplementation during exercise helps performance. Should that practice be banned by the various sport governing bodies? Should sport governing bodies even regulate what is clearly a legal and safe practice?

The purpose of this book, though, is not to address the ethics surrounding supplement use. That's a book unto itself. Certainly in a free country, personal responsibility is paramount and the abuse of supplements (or even food for that matter) is something that no amount of regulation can control. The supplements discussed in this book are limited to those that are legal and can be purchased over the counter by anyone. However, keep in mind that some may be banned by certain sport governing bodies.

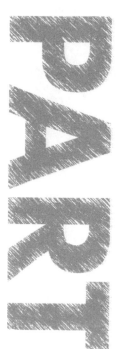

Single Supplements

The study of dietary supplements has grown tremendously in the past decade. An Internet search of the term "dietary supplement" will turn up over 3,600 references! In the world of sports supplements, scientific research is moving at a blistering pace. However, not all supplements are supported with large volumes of data. For instance, there are over 200 studies alone on creatine. And certainly, the scientific evidence is overwhelming that creatine supplementation is safe and effective. On the other hand, a supplement such as boron has little to no data supporting an ergogenic effect.

Although many athletes use combinations of these ingredients, it is still necessary for science to parcel out the effects of single supplements.

Acetyl-L-Carnitine

What Is It?

Acetyl-L-carnitine (ALC) is a molecule composed of acetic acid and the amino acid L-carnitine and is found naturally in the human brain. Interestingly, ALC is sold as a drug in Europe to treat age-related neurological dysfunction, such as Alzheimer's disease and geriatric depression (Pettegrew, Levine, and McClure 2000). The important question, however, is whether it improves athletic performance in strength-power athletes.

How Does It Work?

ALC is supposed to help strength-power athletes via an increase in the male sex hormone testosterone. Testosterone is a potent, anabolic hormone; that is, it helps build tissue, especially skeletal muscle tissue. Theoretically, if one can boost testosterone concentrations in the blood, that person would more easily gain muscle, which would then result in increased strength or power.

The Evidence: Pro or Con?

The ergogenic claims for ALC are mainly based on data using rats. For example, rats in one study were subjected to the stress of cold-water swimming twice daily for 10 days. It was found that giving the rats ALC (dose of 10 mg/day) prevented the normal decrease in blood testosterone in response to the swimming stress (Bidzinska et al. 1993). Rats that did

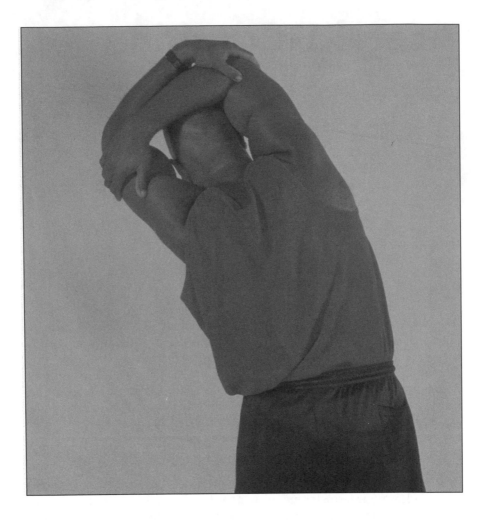

not receive ALC had depressed testosterone concentrations. Unfortunately, there are no studies in humans that show improved strength or power. Though one would suspect that severe stressors might lower blood testosterone, all one could rightly claim for ALC (using very limited evidence) is that it may help maintain normal blood testosterone levels in the face of severe stress.

Guidelines for Use

It isn't clear that strength-power athletes could benefit from ALC supplementation. The only circumstance in which ALC might help is during times of very intense training—for example, two-a-day practices for football players. You could speculate that taking ALC might prevent the drop in testosterone seen with very intense training (which would make for a nice graduate school research project). If athletes were to use ALC assuming that it helps, the equivalent dose (gleaned from data on rats) would be roughly 10 mg per lb of body weight, which would be 2,000 mg for a 200-lb person.

Precautions

In a clinical study performed on elderly humans, a daily dose of 1,500 mg ALC for 90 days had no reported adverse effects (Salvioli and Neri 1994).

Alpha-Ketoglutarate

What Is It?

Alpha-ketoglutarate (AKG) is naturally involved in your body's energy pathways. AKG is an intermediate of the Krebs cycle (a metabolic pathway involved in energy production) and is the precursor for the synthesis of various amino acids, such as glutamine, glutamate, proline, and arginine.

How Does It Work?

AKG is touted as an anti-catabolic, or protein-sparing, agent. That is, if you consume AKG in sufficient amounts, it will prevent the loss of skeletal muscle mass, which often happens after surgery or during a prolonged illness.

The Evidence: Pro or Con?

The evidence for AKG's effectiveness comes from clinical human studies. According to a study from the Department of Anaesthesiology and Intensive Care at the Karolinska Institute in Sweden, the "addition of alpha-ketoglutarate to postoperative total parenteral nutrition prevented the decrease in muscle protein synthesis . . ." (Wernerman, Hammarqvist, and Vinnars 1990). Translation: When doctors infuse high doses of AKG into patients after major surgery, patients lose less muscle mass as a result. Currently, though, there is no evidence that AKG supplementation has any effect on strength-power athletes.

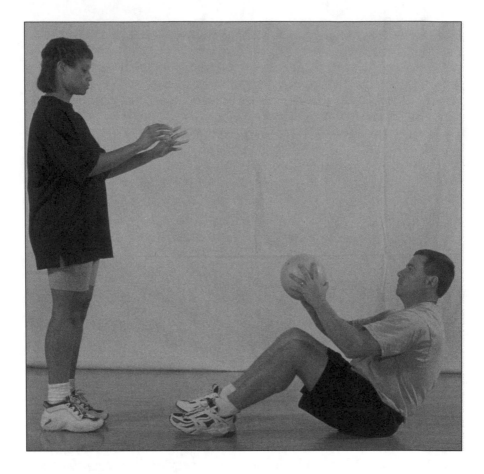

Guidelines for Use

Though AKG has known protein-sparing effects, there is no evidence that it can help strength-power athletes. Also, the dose used is quite high, roughly 20-30 g daily for a 200-lb person (Blomqvist et al. 1995). Thus, AKG, even if it does have a protein-sparing effect, is not a feasible ergogenic aid.

Precautions

Most of the studies performed with AKG have been on patients at postsurgery. Therefore, it would seem reasonable that for those who are healthy, the use of AKG would result in no harmful side effects.

Alpha-Ketoisocaproate

3

What Is It?

Alpha-ketoisocaproate (KIC) is the branched-chain ketoacid derived from the amino acid leucine. KIC administration in growing lambs has been shown to "increase weight gain and muscle growth while decreasing fat deposition" (Flakoll et al. 1991). The truth in humans isn't quite as exciting.

How Does It Work?

KIC has a protein-sparing effect, which means that under certain conditions, taking KIC may help offset the loss of muscle mass. For instance, the infusion of KIC in abdominal surgery patients spared the body's protein nitrogen (Sapir et al. 1983).

The Evidence: Pro or Con?

Although the aforementioned study did find a protein-sparing effect, another study found no such effect in patients with gastrointestinal cancer (Sandstedt, Jorfeldt, and Larsson 1992). Moreover, there is no evidence in humans that supplementation with KIC has a positive effect on performance in strength-power athletes. One could surmise, though, that if KIC truly has a protein-sparing effect, then perhaps it might be useful during times of detraining, when the loss of muscle mass might occur.

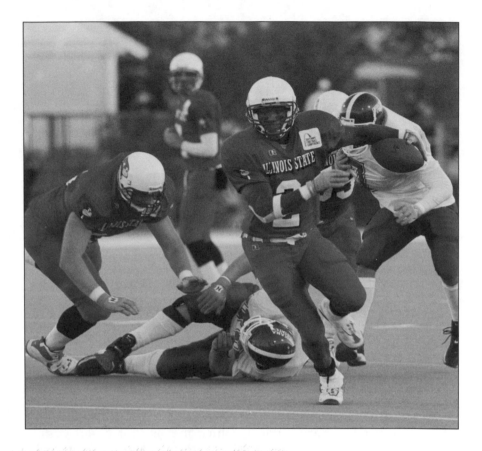

Guidelines for Use

Again, the evidence for KIC's use by strength-power athletes is lacking, and the dosages used in the clinical studies on humans are quite high, 10-20 g daily. Thus, it would be an inconvenient and expensive supplement to consume on a regular basis.

Precautions

Infusion studies in humans show that KIC is well tolerated with no side effects reported, yet one might suspect that the oral ingestion of high doses (>10 g) of KIC might present gastrointestinal problems in certain people.

Androstenedione and Androstenediol

4

What Are They?

Androstenedione (not androstenediol) was made famous by former baseball single-season home run king Mark McGwire. He reluctantly admitted to taking "andro" for the express purpose of helping recovery and improving performance. Whether it actually helped him is debatable. At that time, no studies had been done to test the safety and efficacy of this over-the-counter steroid. So what are androstenedione and androstenediol? Are they steroids? Supplements?

The answer is yes to both. You have probably heard the term *anabolic steroid*, which is the synthetic version of the male hormone testosterone. Anabolic steroids speed up protein synthesis, reduce catabolism, and increase strength and muscle mass in athletes who train with weights, but they also may affect other parts of the body with potential side effects. Anabolic steroids are used primarily by strength-power athletes such as bodybuilders, powerlifters, weightlifters, and sprinters—although they are also likely used by endurance athletes as a way to expedite the postexercise recovery process.

Some scientists call androstenedione and androstenediol (and like compounds) "androgens" or "anabolic-androgenic steroids." Suffice it to say that all of these compounds have a structure similar to testosterone. Structural similarity, however, does not always translate into similar functional effects.

Androstenedione and androstenediol are also commonly referred to as *prohormones*. Because they are the immediate precursors to the male sex hormone testosterone, you'd suspect that they too should exert

11

anabolic effects, assuming they readily convert to testosterone. For instance, if you were to study the metabolic pathway from cholesterol to testosterone—yes, you need cholesterol to make the steroid hormones!—you would see that androstenedione is closer in the metabolic pathway to testosterone than dehydroepiandrosterone (DHEA) is. Does this mean that androstenedione is more anabolic than DHEA? Good question. If mere proximity to testosterone is the answer, then prodigious amounts of cholesterol would have a similar effect as androstenedione, right? Before we jump to this conclusion—and thus run out to load up on bacon cheeseburgers—let's explore the facts and studies.

How Do They Work?

It has been hypothesized that supplementation with these agents should have effects similar to testosterone—that is, having anabolic or muscle-building effects—because of their structural similarity to testosterone and because they can readily convert to testosterone (both prohormones are just one chemical step away from becoming testosterone) (see figure 4.1). If you recall from the endless hours you spent memorizing endocrine physiology—okay, maybe you were spared that torture—you were taught that testosterone (as well as other androgenic hormones) worked by binding to the androgen receptor (AR) in skeletal muscle. Think of receptors as a lock to a door. If you have the correct key (the proper hormone to

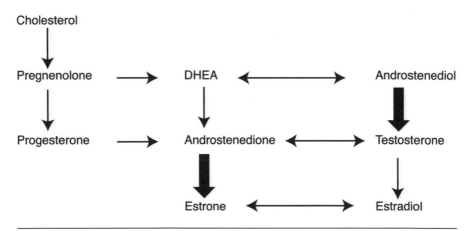

Figure 4.1 Androgen pathways.

open that lock), then you can open this figurative door. When testosterone binds to the AR, it is opening a physiologic door that allows skeletal muscles to produce more protein. This reaction, of course, results in larger overall muscles, and larger muscles should therefore translate into greater strength and power.

The Evidence: Pro or Con?

Research done approximately 40 years ago served as the basis for the marketing campaign used by many supplement companies to sell androstenedione (Mahesh and Greenblatt 1962). In this study, scientists gave two women 100 mg 4-androstenedione orally and found a peak increase (+337%) in total testosterone one hour after ingestion. At 90 minutes, levels had decreased to 50% of the peak. If you know the differences between men and women (not just Mars and Venus stuff), you'd know that women have much lower levels of plasma testosterone to begin with. Therefore, it isn't surprising that you would see such a dramatic rise. Nonetheless, let's examine the current research.

The first questions to ask as we explore this topic are the following: Are there differences between androstenedione and androstenediol, and do either of these compounds actually produce effects similar to testosterone or other anabolic steroids?

Scientists from Iowa State University conducted what is perhaps the best-known (or most highly publicized) study on androstenedione. In an eight-week intervention period, healthy, previously untrained males (aged 19-29 years) were given either a placebo or androstenedione, 300 mg daily each week, except weeks three and six (King et al. 1999). They also engaged in heavy resistance training. In a separate study, scientists studied the effects of a single dose of androstenedione (100 mg) on plasma (blood) concentrations of estrogen (female sex hormone) and testosterone. What did they find?

In the acute study (single dose), the researchers found that a 100 mg dose had no effect on plasma testosterone and estrogen concentrations. In the long-term study, they found no differences in the placebo versus androstenedione group in terms of strength, muscle fiber size, lean body mass, and fat mass. Some of the negative effects of the androstenedione supplementation included a decrease in high-density lipoprotein cholesterol (HDL, also known as the "good" cholesterol) and an increase in serum estradiol and estrone levels (female sex hormones). These changes are probably transient—that is, they revert to normal values on cessation of androstenedione consumption—and there is no evidence at this juncture that androstenedione has any long-term harmful effects.

According to this one study, we can at least say that in untrained, healthy, young males, androstenedione is no better than a placebo in improving muscle strength or size. However, there are several studies that contradict these findings of no acute (short-term) changes in plasma testosterone levels.

For instance, Dr. Conrad Earnest and colleagues (2000) looked at the short-term effects of androstenedione and androstenediol administration on eight young men (aged 24). Each subject ingested a placebo, androstenedione (200 mg), or androstenediol (200 mg), and all subjects underwent all three treatments in a random fashion. Blood was sampled at 30, 60, 90, and 120 minutes after ingestion. Their results showed that androstenedione was better than androstenediol in "the appearance and apparent conversion to total and free testosterone over 90 min . . ." So that means androstenedione is better than androstenediol, right? Well, not so fast.

Dr. Tim Ziegenfuss of Eastern Michigan University examined the effects of a placebo, 100 mg 4-androstenedione, and 100 mg 4-androstenediol (Ziegenfuss and Kerrigan 1999). The 4-androstenedione had no significant effect on total or free testosterone concentrations, but 4-androstenediol produced significant increases in total and free testosterone. At 60 and 90 minutes postingestion, total testosterone increased 40% and 48% and free testosterone increased 29% and 43%.

Regardless, whether androstenedione and androstenediol cause a transient rise in plasma testosterone (or estrogen for that matter) is a minor point. The fundamental question is, does this acute increase in testosterone actually translate into a gain in muscle mass and strength? If it doesn't do either of these, then all this other information is sheer window dressing.

In a recent study appropriately dubbed the "Andro Project," 14 scientists collaborated on an extensive project that sought to determine the short- and long-term effects of androstenedione and androstenediol (Broeder et al. 2000). In this 12-week study, 50 healthy men (aged 35-65) were randomly assigned to either a placebo group, androstenedione group ("dione group," 200 mg daily), or androstenediol group ("diol group," 200 mg daily). Each subject lifted weights three times per week and performed standard resistance exercises. So what happened to these subjects?

With regards to total and free testosterone, there were no changes in baseline levels before and after the treatment. Although figure 4.2 shows that the diol group increased total testosterone, the change was not statistically significant.

However, the hormone levels that did change were plasma estrone and estradiol—both female sex hormones. Figure 4.3 illustrates that in both the dione and diol groups, serum estradiol increased dramatically and

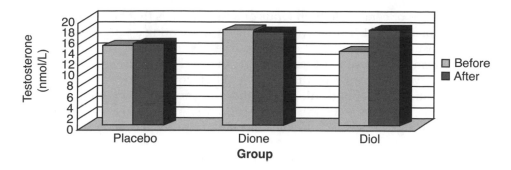

Figure 4.2   Total testosterone. Adapted from Broeder et al. 2000.

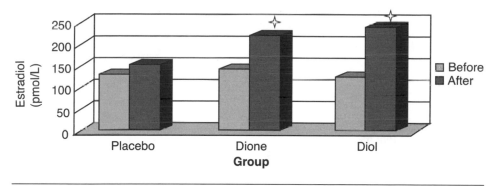

Figure 4.3   Changes in serum estradiol. ✧ = Significant change.

significantly, yet the placebo group did not change to any significant degree. In addition, plasma estrone increased similarly in the dione and diol groups while the control groups demonstrated no significant changes.

The plasma hormone changes are uncompromisingly unimpressive. What about changes in body composition? As shown in figure 4.4, skeletal muscle mass was found to be similar in each group before and after the study.

Muscle strength did not differ among the groups at the conclusion of the study. There was no difference in the increase of the bench press strength (one repetition maximum, or 1-RM) among groups (see figure 4.5). No significant difference was also concluded for leg extension strength.

Perhaps of concern to both kinds of andro users is that both the dione and diol increased "coronary disease risk (representing a 6.5% increase)," as measured by changes in blood lipid levels. However, it is far from convincing that these short-term changes in blood lipids, though negative, have any long-term harmful effects. What you can glean from this information is that both dione and diol are probably no better than a placebo in increasing muscle strength or mass. As far as the significance of the change in plasma hormone and blood lipid levels, only time will tell.

It would be remiss, however, not to mention the one study that showed positive effects of a particular combination of prohormones. In a two-part

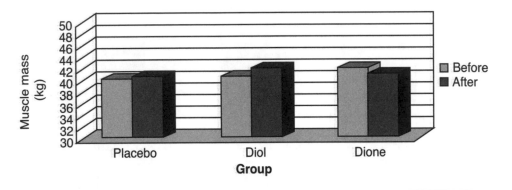

Figure 4.4   Skeletal muscle mass. Adapted from Broeder et al. 2000.

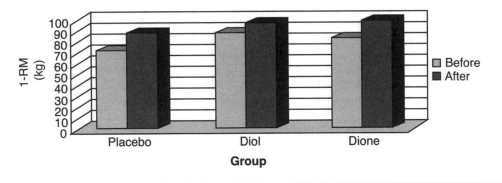

Figure 4.5   Bench press strength, 1-RM. Adapted from Broeder et al. 2000.

study conducted by Dr. Tim Ziegenfuss (Ziegenfuss and Kerrigan 1999), eight men were administered a placebo and various androgens (150 mg). The androgens were composed of the following: 125 mg 4-androstenediol and 5 mg each of 4-androstenedione, 5-androstenedione, 5-androstenediol, 19-nor-4-androstenedione, and 19-nor-5-androstenediol. Obviously, most of the supplement is 4-androstenediol (83%). It is interesting to note that this prohormone was consumed as a sublingual preparation—that is, the dose was administered by placing it under the tongue—in the hopes of improving the delivery of the hormones to the blood and thus bypassing the liver. They found that the acute oral consumption of this combination produced an increase in total testosterone that peaked at 40 minutes, a 98% increase. By 180 minutes, values returned to baseline.

More important, Dr. Ziegenfuss examined the effects of a much higher dose of the same sublingual prohormone combination. Fourteen recreationally active, eugonadal men (approximately 24 years old) were given daily for four weeks either a placebo or the prohormone (450 mg). The prohormone-supplemented group had significant increases in body weight (3.96 lb, or 2.3%), fat-free mass (1.76 lb, 1.1%), vertical jump (2.0 in, 9.3%), total body water (5.4 l, 10.5%), and extracellular fluid volume (2.3 l, 11.8%). The placebo group had no changes in any of these levels. There were also no changes for either group in basal hormone concentrations (testosterone, estradiol, luteinizing hormone), which would suggest that there was no negative feedback effect on the hypothalamic-pituitary-gonadal axis. (*Note:* This is in contrast to the study by Dr. Broeder in which he found that androstenedione caused a drop in luteinizing hormone levels, which would signify a negative effect on hypothalamic-pituitary function.) In addition, there was no change in either group for blood lipids or organ function. Unexpectedly (and inexplicably) high-density lipoprotein cholesterol (HDL-C) levels increased in the placebo and prohormone group.

Guidelines for Use

Most of the scientific literature on androstenedione shows no effect on strength, power, or muscle size. These conclusions could be due to inadequate dosages, insufficient duration of use, or because it just doesn't work. Although the study by Dr. Broeder showed no effect in middle-aged men, perhaps it might help the elderly who have low levels of testosterone. Another possibility might be that women—who have low plasma testosterone to begin with, an average of about 8-10% of the normal adult male—may incur the most benefit from supplementing with androstenedione or androstenediol (see table 4.1). Alternatively, taking androstenedione acutely to promote a transient rise in testosterone might

Table 4.1 Normal Range of Plasma Testosterone		
Male	300-1,200 ng/dl	10.5-42.0 nmol/L
Female	30-95 ng/dl	1.0-3.0 nmol/L

have some sort of ergogenic effect. For a young male with normal testosterone levels, it is likely that androstenedione has no effect on muscle strength or size.

With regards to androstenediol, Broeder et al. (2000) found no effect of its use in middle-aged men. The only study that resulted in any sort of effect used moderately high doses (450 mg daily) and a different method of delivery (sublingually). We can surmise then that if it has no effect on middle-aged men, then it probably has no effect on young men. Of course, the limitations of these studies (and most dietary supplement studies) are the dosages used, the populations studied, and the duration of treatments. From the existing research, it appears that to see any sort of ergogenic effect, older men or women would be the best populations to study.

Precautions

There is evidence that you may experience a negative alteration in blood lipids and plasma hormone levels. For example, your HDL could go down; your plasma estrogen could go up (which is not good for men); or there may be a drop in your luteinizing hormone. It isn't known, though, if these changes are of physiological significance because the treatment period in most of these studies was three months or less. As a footnote, both of these prohormones are on the International Olympic Committee's banned substance list despite the fact that there is no evidence that either is anabolic or has ergogenic effects.

β-Hydroxy-β-Methylbutyrate

What Is It?

β-Hydroxy-β-Methylbutyrate (HMB) is a breakdown product (metabolite) of the amino acid leucine (Nissen, Sharp et al. 1996). Leucine is an essential building block of protein in all tissues, and it is found in all dietary protein. Among the amino acids, leucine holds a special place: In addition to being an essential amino acid (one that must be supplied from the diet), it's also one of three branched chain amino amino acids (the other two are valine and isoleucine). But what ultimately separates leucine as being unique is its role in regulating protein synthesis and protein breakdown.

How Does It Work?

The first understanding of what effect HMB has on protein metabolism was research that showed the first metabolite of leucine, called ketoisocaproate (KIC), duplicating most, if not all, of the effects of leucine in tissues. Early research (Chua, Siehl, and Morgan 1979; Mortimore et al. 1987) found that both leucine and KIC decreased proteolysis (protein breakdown) and increased protein synthesis in isolated tissues. Additional studies found nitrogen sparing (Cerosimo et al. 1983; Mortimore et al. 1987; Mitch, Walser, and Spair 1981) and reductions in muscle glucose utilization (Buckspan et al. 1986) with KIC in humans subjected to stressful situations. The doses of leucine used in these studies were about 120 g per day (Cerosimo et al. 1983) and about half that for KIC (Buckspan et al. 1986; Mitch, Walser, and Spair 1981). Furthermore, it must be pointed out that most of theses studies were conducted under extreme conditions, such as starvation, trauma, or severe burns.

The data with KIC, however, indicated that the leucine effect was not due to leucine but instead due to a downstream product. Thus, the same question remained: Was the effect due to KIC or some further breakdown product in the pathway of which there are about eight additional biochemicals? In the early 1980s, scientists suggested an alternative metabolic pathway of leucine metabolism that indicated that KIC was metabolized by an enzyme distinct to HMB (figure 5.1). Scientists at Iowa State University were the first to test the hypothesis that this HMB metabolite may mediate the effects of leucine and KIC on protein metabolism. Their postulation led them first to a series of animal experiments and later to humans spanning the last 10 years. These extensive studies indicate that HMB is the bioactive component of leucine

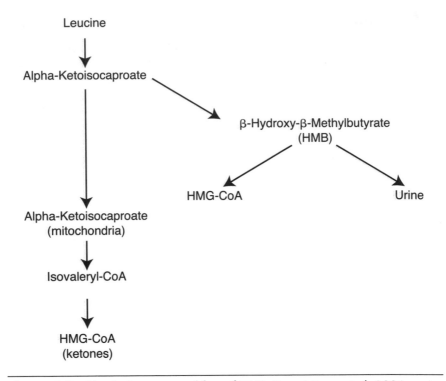

Figure 5.1 Metabolic origin and fate of HMB. From Nissen et al. 1996.

metabolism that plays a regulator role in protein metabolism (Nissen, Panton et al. 1996; Nissen, Sharp et al. 1996).

Research in animals suggests that HMB plays some role in protein metabolism, especially in stressful situations. Although no one is certain of the mechanism(s) behind HMB, scientists have been working on two hypotheses (Nissen, Sharp et al. 1996).

Hypothesis 1: HMB may be an essential component of the cell membrane. Scientists propose that under stressful situations, the body may not make enough HMB to satisfy the increased needs of tissues. It could also be that stress may alter enzymes or concentration of certain biochemicals that decrease normal HMB production. Either scenario requires dietary supplementation of HMB for skeletal muscle system to function maximally.

Hypothesis 2: HMB may regulate enzymes responsible for muscle tissue breakdown. This theory is supported by the evidence found in several studies where biochemical indicators of muscle damage (CPK and 3-MH) decreased (see "The Evidence" section for an explanation).

The Evidence: Pro or Con?

The first human-performance study with HMB was conducted by Dr. Nissen and colleagues at Iowa State university (Nissen, Sharp et al. 1996). In this study, male subjects participated in a resistance-training program and were assigned to either a control group, a group that consumed 1.5 g HMB per day, or a group that consumed 3 g HMB per day. After a one-week adaptation period, the three-week supplementation and exercise protocol (total body weight-training program) started. After only one week of training and supplementation, muscle protein breakdown in the group given 3 g HMB decreased 44% (compared with the placebo group) as measured by 3-methylhistidine (3-MH) loss in urine. (3-MH is a muscle-specific amino acid that is produced and lost in urine only when muscle protein is broken down.) Muscle protein breakdown continued to be lower in the HMB group for the entire three-week study. A second indicator of muscle damage and muscle breakdown is the muscle-specific enzyme called creatine phosphokinase (CPK). This enzyme was also markedly decreased with HMB supplementation.

The biochemical indicators of muscle damage were also accompanied by increases in muscle strength (total weight lifted) for both of the HMB-supplemented groups: 23% for 1.5 g and 29% for 3 g. This initial study then indicates that HMB may reduce the damaging effects of resistance exercise on muscle with the net result being maximal strength increase in response to exercise. In agreement, several studies have demonstrated positive gains in strength in both men and woman (aged 18-70) from supplementing 3 g HMB/day while on a weight-training program (Gallagher et al. 2000a; Nissen et al. 1997; Panton et al. 2000; Vukovich et al. 1997). These findings suggest that supplementation with 1.5 to 3 g HMB per day may augment training-induced changes in strength in untrained men and women.

In contrast, the effects of HMB supplementation during resistance training in well-trained athletes are equivocal. While Dr. Nissen and colleagues (1996) did demonstrate positive effects with HMB supplementation in football players, Dr. Kreider and colleagues at the University of Memphis have reported no beneficial effects in well-trained athletes (Almada et al. 1997; Kreider et al. 1997; Kreider et al. 1999). Therefore, more research is needed to validate whether HMB supplementation would enhance the training adaptations of exercise for well-trained athletes.

The effects of HMB on lean body mass are promising. Kreider et al. (1999) found that 3 or 6 g per day of HMB supplementation did not affect training-induced changes in body composition; however, Vukovich, Stubbs, and Bohlken (2001) found that HMB supplementation tended to increase fat-free mass in 70-year-old adults participating in a strength-training program.

In an extensive study done at East Tennessee University (Panton et al. 2000), scientists studied the effects of resistance training plus HMB supplementation on 39 men and 36 women between the ages of 20 and 40. All subjects trained three times per week for four weeks and were supplemented with 3.0 g HMB per day or a placebo. They found that the HMB group had greater gains in strength and lean body mass (see figure 5.2). According to these investigators, "This study showed, regardless of gender or training status, HMB may increase upper body strength and minimize muscle damage when combined with an exercise program."

Guidelines for Use

As you can see, HMB is a very intriguing dietary supplement that may benefit the strength and power athlete. Further research will confirm the adaptive response of the athlete who supplements with HMB. An effective dose appears to be 1.5 to 3 g per day (Gallagher et al. 2000a; Nissen et al. 1997; Panton et al. 2000; Vukovich et al. 1997).

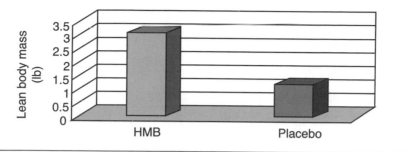

Figure 5.2 Changes in lean body mass after HMB supplementation.

Precautions

Studies ranging in length from one to eight weeks have demonstrated up to 6 g HMB per day is safe and well tolerated (Gallagher et al. 2000b; Nissen et al. 2000). An examination of the studies that used at least a dose of 3 g HMB per day, for a three- to eight-week duration—males and females, young and old, exercising or nonexercising—have all demonstrated no harmful side effects of HMB on organ, tissue, and blood markers of health. In fact, HMB may even help improve cardiovascular health.

Boron

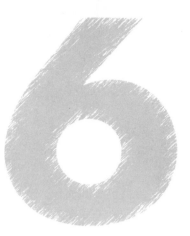

What Is It?

Boron is a trace mineral that is essential for proper utilization of calcium. According to scientists at the National Research Council (1989), boron "appears to affect calcium and magnesium metabolism and may be needed for membrane function." It is interesting to note, though, that according to Ferrando and Green (1993), "boron essentiality in humans has not been established."

How Does It Work?

Boron can supposedly increase plasma concentrations of testosterone. By promoting a rise in this anabolic hormone, boron should theoretically produce a gain in muscle mass and strength.

The Evidence: Pro or Con?

There are no studies that demonstrate a positive ergogenic effect of boron. For instance, Ferrando and Green (1993) studied 19 male bodybuilders, aged 20-27. Of those, 10 were given 2.5 mg boron daily while the others received a placebo. All subjects participated in a weight-training program during the seven-week intervention. At the conclusion of the study, there were no differences between the two groups' body composition or strength (see figure 6.1).

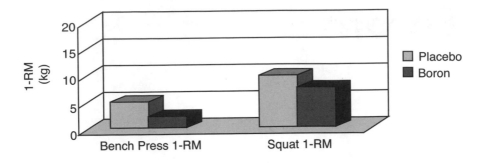

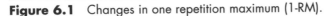

Figure 6.1   Changes in one repetition maximum (1-RM).

Guidelines for Use

It isn't clear that boron supplementation is justified. Though you might find some utility if you are deficient in boron intake, at this point we do not recommend supplementation.

Precautions

Low boron intake may negatively affect hand-eye coordination and manual dexterity (Wolinsky 1998). Boron supplementation of 3 mg per day for one year in female college athletes and sedentary people produced a rise in serum magnesium levels, whereas urinary calcium losses increased over time.

Branched-Chain Amino Acids

What Are They?

The branched-chain amino acids (BCAA) consist of valine, leucine, and isoleucine. BCAA are found in high concentrations in skeletal muscle and are an integral part of muscle metabolism. This section focuses on the combination of the three amino acids as well as the single amino acid leucine.

How Do They Work?

The BCAA have a variety of functions. First, they are involved in the synthesis of glutamine in skeletal muscle. Glutamine (see pages 61-66) is an important amino acid, particularly during times of stress. Second, BCAA can be used as a fuel source, and there is also evidence that indicates a possible anti-catabolic or protein-sparing effect.

The Evidence: Pro or Con?

Though BCAA supplementation is generally targeted toward strength-power athletes, particularly bodybuilders, much of the research has been done on endurance athletes. Our focus is on its effects (or lack thereof) on strength-power athletes. Unfortunately, there are no studies that suggest an ergogenic effect of BCAA supplementation in strength-power athletes; however, there is related work that may show how BCAA supplementation could affect strength-power athletes.

For example, in a study in which 16 subjects participated in a 21-day trek at an altitude of 3,255 meters (10,679 feet), subjects received daily either a placebo or 11.5 g BCAA (5.76 g leucine, 2.88 g isoleucine, and 2.88 g valine) (Schena et al. 1992). During the trek, caloric intake decreased by 4% in both groups, and both groups lost a similar amount of body weight and fat. However, lean body mass improved in the BCAA group (+1.5%) with no change in the placebo group. Of interest to strength-power athletes, lower-limb maximal power decreased less in the BCAA group than in the placebo group (-2.4% vs. -7.8%). Furthermore, arm muscle cross-sectional area did not change in the BCAA group, yet the placebo group experienced a 6.8% decrease.

In a similar study, Bigard et al. (1996) examined 24 highly trained subjects who participated in six consecutive sessions of ski mountaineering, with six to eight hours per session at 2,500 to 4,100 meters altitude (8,202 to 13,452 feet). The subjects ingested daily 22.4 g BCAA (7.8 g leucine, 3.4 g isoleucine, 11.2 g valine) or a carbohydrate placebo. Body weight decreased significantly in the placebo group but not in the BCAA group, but there were no differences in fat and lean body mass between groups. Interestingly, peak power measured during an incremental bicycle exercise decreased in the placebo group but not in the BCAA group. Knee extensor maximal voluntary contraction (MVC) strength (isometric) was not different between groups.

So in essence, they found no differences in fat mass and lean body mass and no differences in maximal leg strength. Peak power, however, tended to decrease less in the BCAA group. What exactly does all of this mean? It isn't clear at the moment, and other studies continue to add to the list of unresolved issues.

For instance, in one study, 30 days of daily supplementation with 14 g BCAA (50% leucine, 25% valine, and 25% isoleucine) in a group of healthy, untrained subjects resulted in a slight but significant increase in fat-free mass (+1.3%) and grip strength (+8.1%) (Candeloro et al. 1995). The relevance of an 8.1% increase in grip strength is questionable. Nonetheless, these studies do suggest that BCAA may ameliorate the loss of strength, and though remote, another possibility is that it may actually increase strength.

But what about the single amino acid leucine? According to work from the University of Jyvaskyla in Finland, "its [leucine] oxidation rate is higher than that of valine or isoleucine. Leucine also stimulates protein synthesis in muscle . . ." (Mero 1999). The theoretical aspects of leucine supplementation are definitely intriguing as well, yet only one study has examined the use of leucine in strength-power athletes (Mero et al. 1997). In this investigation, 20 male track and field power athletes were given leucine or placebo tablets. The daily dosage was 50 mg/kg body weight (22.7 mg/lb, or approximately 4.5 g leucine daily for a 200-lb person). They found that during 10 weeks of intense training, serum leucine concentration decreased 20.1% in the placebo group during the first 5 weeks of training but stabilized during the last 5 weeks. Conversely, when leucine was supplemented, there were no changes in serum leucine concentration; however, levels of all amino acids combined decreased (in the blood) in both groups. Additionally, in both groups serum testosterone and cortisol increased during the first 5 weeks, yet during the second 5 weeks, only testosterone dropped. What can be gleaned from this study is that taking leucine helps prevent a drop in serum (blood) leucine. The results do not indicate that taking leucine improved strength or power in any of these athletes.

Guidelines for Use

There is only one study that has examined the role of BCAA or leucine on strength-power athletes (and that study dealt with leucine only). Basically, you are left to your best guess as to how to supplement with the BCAA or leucine. The evidence for BCAA and leucine is at the moment equivocal

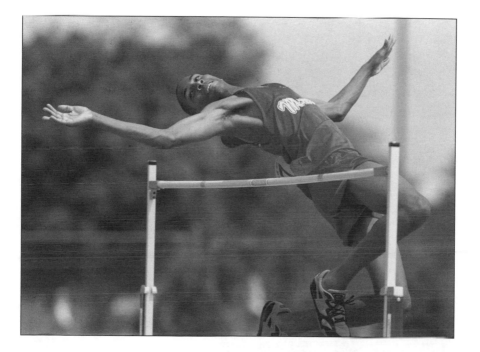

with regards to endurance performance. If athletes were to choose these as dietary supplements, they could use the daily dosages used in scientific investigations: 4-5 g leucine and 14 g BCAA (50% leucine, 25% valine, and 25% isoleucine). A trial-and-error approach with these dosages might serve as a useful start to see if they indeed have ergogenic effects.

Precautions

For high-dose BCAA or leucine consumption, there are no known harmful side effects. Because these substances are acids, though, some people may experience gastrointestinal distress.

Caffeine

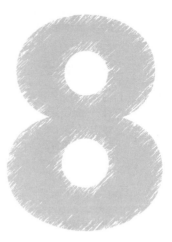

What Is It?

The effects of caffeine have been known for quite some time. For instance, coffee, one of the most widely consumed caffeinated foods, originated in Africa circa A.D. 575. But what exactly is it? Caffeine is an alkaloid, and it is also found in tea, chocolate, cola drinks, and various over-the-counter medications. Although it is touted as an endurance-performance aid, its effect on the central nervous system may have an ergogenic effect on strength- or power-related activities.

How Does It Work?

There are several possibilities that explain the performance-enhancing effect of caffeine. The traditional hypothesis is that caffeine increases the levels of hormones such as epinephrine and norepinephrine, also known as the catecholamines. The catecholamines promote fat utilization and result in the sparing of intramuscular glycogen. This effect, though, would be more important during prolonged endurance exercises; how caffeine might affect strength or power-type exercises is currently unknown. One possible ergogenic effect is that caffeine can increase one's ability to maximally activate skeletal muscle fibers (Kalmar and Cafarelli 1999).

The Evidence: Pro or Con?

In a study published in the *British Journal of Sports Medicine* (Williams et al. 1988), subjects ingested 7 mg caffeine per kg body weight (about 3.2 mg per lb, or 640 mg for a 200-lb person). An hour after ingestion, they performed 15-second maximal exercise bouts on a cycle ergometer, and it was later concluded that the caffeine supplement had no effect on peak power or total work. In another study (Collomp et al. 1991), 5 mg caffeine per kg body weight (approximately 2.3/lb, or 460 mg for a 200-lb person) was no better than a placebo during a 30-second cycle ergometer sprint test (a Wingate test). Other studies (Greer, McLean, and Graham 1998; Vanakoski et al. 1998) have shown no effect of higher doses of caffeine—6-7 mg/kg (2.7-3.6 mg/lb) body weight—on high-intensity, short-duration exercise.

However, a couple of studies that do demonstrate an ergogenic effect of caffeine during anaerobic exercise are worth noting. In one study, 14 subjects ingested either a placebo or 250 mg caffeine in a random order and double-blind fashion (Anselme et al. 1992). Caffeine increased maximal anaerobic power (+7%) in comparison with the placebo. In another study, the same dose of caffeine (250 mg) was given to trained and untrained swimmers (Collomp et al. 1992). Anaerobic power was determined by the mean sprint swimming speed during 100 m sprints. Trained swimmers only experienced an improvement in sprint swimming speed as a result of caffeine ingestion. It isn't clear why untrained subjects didn't experience a similar effect.

Guidelines for Use

Even though caffeine supplementation can lengthen time before exhaustion during endurance events, the evidence for an ergogenic effect during strength-power type events isn't strong. Several studies show no effect of caffeine while a minority of studies show a positive effect. Differences in subject population (e.g., trained vs. untrained, caffeine users vs. nonusers) may affect the results of these studies. Because each of us has an individual response that is not identical to a group average, it would be hard to predict if you are caffeine responsive or not. Certainly, the mild stimulant effect of caffeine on the central nervous system may make it a worthwhile preworkout supplement. The upper limit you'd want to consume is a dose of 6 mg per kg body weight (545 mg for a 200-lb person), which approaches the legal limit set by the International Olympic Committee. Perhaps consuming caffeine 60 minutes before exercise may confer a performance-enhancing effect. See figure 8.1 for the caffeine content of some commonly consumed products.

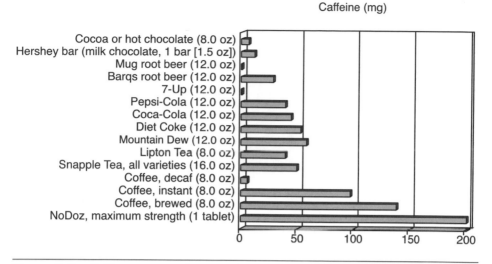

Figure 8.1 Caffeine content of commonly consumed products. Adapted from National Coffee Association et al. 1996.

Precautions

Excessive (>250-300 mg) ingestion may result in caffeine "intoxication," which depends in part on each person's sensitivity to caffeine. Habitual caffeine consumers may find that much higher doses result in intoxication while nonusers may find a single dose of caffeine to be problematic. Common symptoms include restlessness, nervousness, insomnia, excitement, gastrointestinal distress, muscle twitching, rambling flow of thought and speech, tachycardia (rapid heart rate), and psychomotor agitation.

Nonetheless, moderate use of caffeine is entirely safe and should not pose a health risk to active people. In fact, the FDA classified caffeine in 1958 as "generally recognized as safe" (GRAS).

Carbohydrate

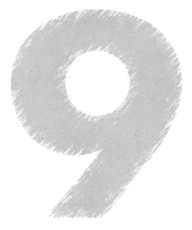

What Is It?

Carbohydrates are also known as starches or sugars. They can be divided into the following groups: monosaccharides—one sugar molecule, such as fructose and glucose; disaccharides—two sugar molecules linked together, such as sucrose or table sugar (glucose plus fructose); oligosaccharides—three to nine sugar molecules linked together, such as those found in legumes; and polysaccharides—ten to thousands of sugar links such as starches and fiber.

How Does It Work?

Because carbohydrates serve as the primary fuel source for high-intensity exercise, it would make sense that consuming sufficient amounts is necessary for optimal exercise performance. For instance, your average 80 kg person (176 lb) stores approximately 400 g glycogen in his skeletal muscles and 100 g in the liver. That 400 g glycogen might last—if you're lucky—a couple hours of continuous exercise. But does intense weight training increase your body's requirement for this important fuel? Let's consider some of the known evidence.

The Evidence: Pro or Con?

In a study from Texas Christian University at Fort Worth, scientists looked at the effects of a pre-exercise carbohydrate diet on weight-lifting performance (Mitchell et al. 1997). Eleven resistance-trained men (average

age 24 years) first performed bicycle exercise to deplete the glycogen stores of quadriceps femoris muscles (large front thigh muscles). For the next two days, one group consumed a low-carbohydrate diet—0.37 g carbohydrate/kg body weight, about 0.17 g/lb (34 g for a 200-lb person)—and the other group consumed a high-carbohydrate diet—7.66 g carbohydrate/kg body weight, or 3.48/lb (about 696 g for a 200-lb person). The results? As measured in repetitions multiplied by weight lifted, researchers found no difference in performance for the squat, leg press, or knee extension.

In another study, Dalton and colleagues (1999) found that consumption of carbohydrates, taken 30 minutes before the test, did not affect leg extensions and bench press exercise performance—that is, 80% of 10 repetitions maximum (10-RM) done to momentary muscular failure.

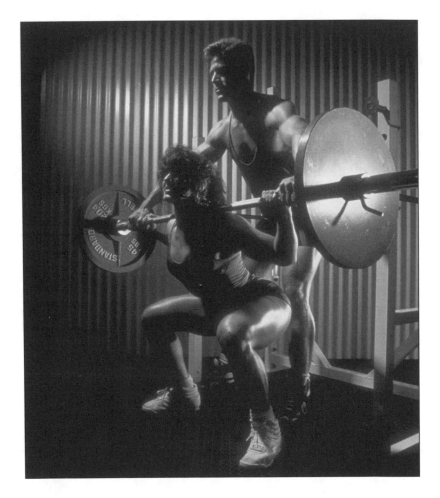

Guidelines for Use

Science doesn't seem to support the ingestion of either a high-carbohydrate diet or the acute consumption of carbohydrates before a resistance exercise bout. With that in mind, we do know that intramuscular carbohydrates (i.e., glycogen) do serve as the primary fuel source during resistance exercises. Though strength-power athletes do not need the amount of carbohydrates (per kg body weight) that an endurance athlete would, it would be unwise for strength-power athletes to purposely restrict carbohydrate consumption. As long as strength-power athletes consume nutrient-dense carbohydrates, like brown rice and whole wheat bread, as part of their everyday eating habits—and not "load up on carbs" as endurance athletes do—their performance should not be adversely affected.

Precautions

Though individual responses might dictate what an athlete does regarding carbohydrate consumption, one word of caution is to avoid high-glycemic carbohydrates about 30-60 minutes before resistance training. High-glycemic carbohydrates elicit a quick rise in blood glucose and therefore in plasma insulin. In turn, the rise in insulin may result in a transient hypoglycemic effect (low blood sugar), which could adversely affect exercise performance. Examples of high-glycemic carbohydrates are glucose, white rice, white bread, and new potatoes.

Chromium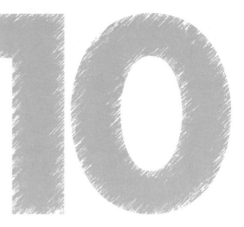

What Is It?

Chromium is an essential trace mineral found in the typical American diet. The most widely used chromium supplement is called chromium picolinate. Picolinate is a special chemical substance, called a chelator, which plays an important role in the delivery of minerals, including chromium, to places in the body where they are needed (Evans 1996).

How Does It Work?

The presence of chromium may act as a cofactor for insulin. Chromium amplifies its actions and thus enhances the efficiency of insulin's effects on glucose, amino acids, and fatty acid flux into the cell with subsequent glycogen, protein, and triglyceride synthesis (Lefavi et al. 1992). In other words, chromium helps drive nutrients such as glucose, amino acids, and fats into your cells.

The Evidence: Pro or Con?

Dr. Clancy and colleagues (1994) tested the effects of chromium on sprint power and dynamic strength. Thirty-six football players engaged in their regular preseason training and supplemented with either a chromium supplement or a placebo for nine weeks. The results showed that despite the increase in chromium intake, there were no significant gains in sprint power or strength. Although the athletes engaged in strenuous physical activity, which has been shown to increase the excretion of chromium, it is likely that none were near chromium deficiency or depletion. The average caloric intake per day for the football players was around 3,752 kcal. According to Lukaski and colleagues (1996), for every 1,000 kcal, there is an estimated 15 mcg of chromium. The caloric consumption per day in the Clancy study is far above the norm and would likely lead to a higher level of chromium than the average person would consume. Therefore, the high-calorie diet would decrease the need for any chromium supplementation.

But let's examine the Lukaski study a little more closely. Dr. Lukaski and colleagues studied a population that would be more likely to be chromium deficient. The subjects were 36 men, aged 19 to 29, who were not actively involved with physical training before the study. During the study, the subjects engaged in eight weeks of moderate weight training while supplementing with either chromium or a placebo. The purpose of the study was to determine if the chromium-supplemented group would increase strength significantly more than the placebo group. There were a couple of notable issues with the study, though. Dietary analyses indicated

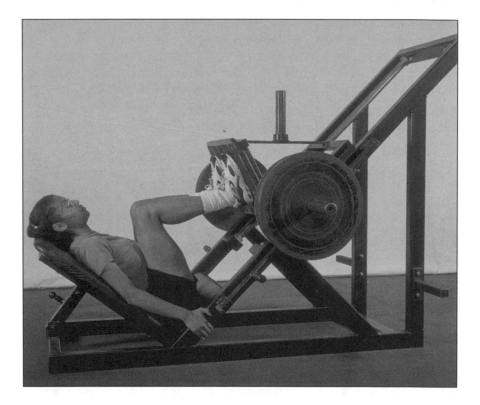

that chromium intake for the majority of the group was slightly less than the daily recommendation. In addition, the weight training may have increased the excretion rates of chromium, thereby increasing the need for chromium supplementation.

The findings were that both groups increased strength significantly, yet there was no significant difference between the chromium-supplemented group and the placebo group. Dr. Lukaski reported that the average caloric intake for these subjects was around 3,000 kcal per day, which equates to 45 mcg of chromium, close to the minimum recommended requirement. Although the caloric intake in this study was significantly lower than what Dr. Clancy reported, the subjects were still far from chromium depletion.

It is important to remember that chromium supplementation serves as a preventive method for chromium depletion. In the previous studies, the likelihood of the subjects being chromium-depleted was not significantly high. In 1998, Dr. Walker and colleagues examined a population that was more likely to be chromium-deficient. In this study, 20 college male wrestlers were put into a control group, a chromium-supplemented group, or a placebo group during the final 16 weeks of preseason training. The wrestlers were tested for their maximum strength and power in the bench and leg press. The results indicated that chromium supplementation did not increase strength or power in wrestlers who were likely to be chromium deficient. In fact, Dr. Walker reported that the average muscular strength and power of the chromium-supplemented group slightly decreased, unlike the placebo and the control groups who showed a slight increase in both muscular strength and power.

Guidelines for Use

The recommended intake of chromium is 50 to 200 mcg per day. It would appear that most if not all Americans eating sufficient calories obtain enough chromium from diet alone. Those athletes that are on low-calorie diets and are training hard for an extended period may want to consider supplementing chromium in their diet.

Precautions

Also, chromium may compete with iron at the binding sites of serum proteins. This preliminary conclusion suggests that the continued supplementation of chromium with picolinic acid—coupled with the evidence of altered iron metabolism in the presence of picolinic acid, particularly in high doses—may result in iron deficiency.

Colostrum

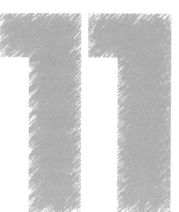

What Is It?

Milk is a great source of protein and other nutrients such as calcium and vitamin D. It is also, of course, our first nourishment in the first days of life. But, in the first 24 to 72 hours, when we undergo a period of rapid development, we are actually supported by a special type of mother's milk called colostrum. It is the first mammary secretion provided for newborns, and it occurs just before the onset of genuine lactation.

The formulation of colostrum is much more complex than simple milk; its components are not found in such high concentrations anywhere else in nature (Kishikawa et al. 1996; Kuhne et al. 2000). There are several major components to colostrum, two of which are currently undergoing vigorous investigation: The growth factor fraction (IGF-1) and the immunoglobulin fraction. A third remaining fraction contains enzymes, proteins, various peptides, and other compounds of lesser interest to athletes (Mero et al. 1997; Pakkanen and Aalto 1997).

How Does It Work?

There is evidence to suggest that the IGF-1 in colostrum may stimulate cellular (muscle) growth (Kishikawa et al. 1996; Kuhne et al. 2000). The current hypothesis is that the combination of high quality proteins and

IGF-1 found in colostrum may optimally stimulate muscle building and thus strength and power (Buckley et al. 2001).

The Evidence: Pro or Con?

In a double blind, placebo-controlled study—neither athletes nor researchers knew who was getting colostrum or placebo—39 fit, young men (aged 18-35) completed an eight-week running program, running three times a week for 45 minutes per session (Buckley et al. 1998). They consumed 60 g per day of either colostrum or a placebo (whey protein). At the start, and again at the fourth and eighth weeks, all subjects did two treadmill runs to exhaustion, with 20 minutes rest between runs. At the beginning of the study, no differences existed in treadmill running performance. At week four, both groups had improved similarly in treadmill running performance. At week eight, the colostrum group ran farther than the placebo group: 4,662 m vs. 4,237 m, a 10% difference.

Furthermore, the colostrum-supplemented group showed a trend toward reduced serum creatine kinase levels. Creatine kinase is a critically important muscle-cell enzyme, which some experts believe can be used as a marker of muscle-cell damage. If blood creatine kinase concentrations rocket upward, it's often a sign that significant muscle damage has occurred. On the other hand, if creatine kinase levels stay fairly normal, some researchers believe that an individual has not experienced much muscle trauma.

Both groups lost body fat, but the colostrum-fed group lost slightly more, 1.8 lb vs. 1.5 lb. Dietary analysis of the two groups showed no differences in dietary intake. So colostrum, in combination with a mild running program, appears to slightly improve performance, potentially reduce muscle breakdown, and augment the loss of body fat.

Another recent double-blind, placebo-controlled study investigated the effects of supplementation with colostrum (Smeets et al. 2000). The subjects were a group of elite female and male field hockey players, including players from the Dutch national team. All subjects consumed either 60 g colostrum protein powder or whey protein powder per day (the latter a placebo) during the first eight weeks of competition season. Researchers examined the functional high muscle power output (5 · 10 m sprint and vertical jump) and endurance running during the eight weeks of supplementation. The endurance tests demonstrated that there were no significant differences between the colostrum group and the whey group; however, the colostrum group had significantly better improvement in

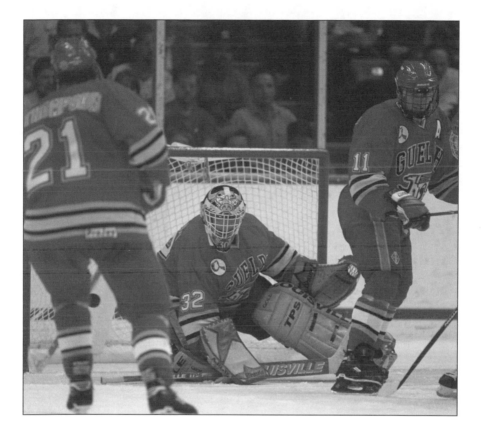

the 5 · 10 m sprint test, and there was a strong trend for a better improvement in jump performance in the colostrum group. Therefore, we can conclude from this study that in elite field hockey players, colostrum supplementation does seem to improve performance in high muscle power output better than whey. With endurance-type exercises, there appears to be no difference in improvement between the two groups.

Guideline for Use

The recommended dose is 60 g per day based on the available data on performance. However, work done by Antonio, Sanders, and Van Gammeren (2001) showed that a 20 g per day dose during an eight-week period for those who exercised regularly resulted in a significant gain in lean body mass even though performance did not change (see figure 11.1).

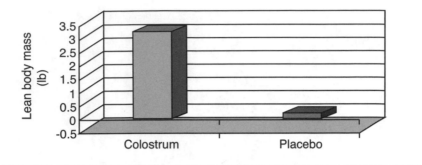

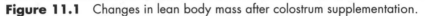

Figure 11.1 Changes in lean body mass after colostrum supplementation.

Precautions

Colostrum contains a wide range of growth promoting factors. One could argue that it has an effect on doping-related testing. However, a study was performed in which human growth hormone, IGF-1 levels, and hematocrit were measured in the blood before and after four weeks of supplementation (60 g/day) (Kuipers et al. 2001). The results demonstrated that none of the parameters changed, and the doping test was negative.

Creatine

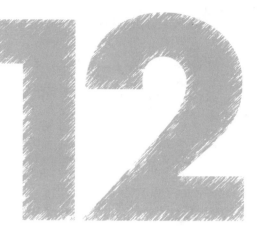

What Is It?

Creatine (Cr) is a nitrogenous organic compound that is synthesized to a small extent (2%) in the liver, pancreas, and kidneys from the amino acids arginine, methionine and glycine (Pearson et al. 1999). Creatine can also be obtained through exogenous sources, such as high-protein foods like fish and beef (see table 12.1) (Williams, Kreider, and Branch 1999). Approximately 95% of all the creatine stores in the body are found in skeletal muscle.

Table 12.1 Creatine Content in Select Food

Food	Grams Cr/lb	Grams Cr/kg
Cod	1.4	3.0
Beef	2.0	4.5
Herring	3.0-4.5	6.5-10.0
Milk	0.05	0.1
Pork	2.3	5.0
Salmon	2.0	4.5
Shrimp	trace	trace
Tuna	1.8	4.0

Adapted, by permission, from M.H. Williams, M.R. Kreider, and D. Branch, 1999, *Creatine: The power supplement,* (Champaign, IL: Human Kinetics), 15.

How Does It Work?

The human body relies on three main metabolic systems for energy, either by direct means from the adenosine triphosphate–phosphocreatine (ATP-PCr) system or indirectly through aerobic and anaerobic glycolysis. The breakdown of adenosine triphosphate (ATP) is how your body produces energy, and phosphocreatine (PCr) is a way of helping regenerate ATP. The ATP-PCr system is always the first to respond to exercise. A drawback to the quick energy and accessibility of phosphocreatine or creatine phosphate (CP) is its rapid depletion (Gilliam et al. 2000). The depletion of the PCr stores occurs at an extremely fast rate; less than 15 seconds (Edwards et al. 2000).

It was this decreased synthesis of energy (ATP) that brought about the notion that creatine supplementation may be a means of increasing PCr and creatine stores, thus reducing fatigue and increasing performance (Pearson et al. 1999). Demant and Rhodes (1999) reported that Cr supplementation of 20 to 30 g per day for three days or longer is believed to enhance exercise performance in two ways. First, Cr may provide a greater initial source of energy by increasing the initial amounts of PCr in the muscle. Second, providing more free Cr aids the rate of PCr regeneration during recovery. A third possible mechanism is an increase in protein synthesis rate by greater satellite cell activity. Satellite cells are located on muscle cell membranes, and increased satellite cell activity repairs damaged muscle fibers, enlarges existing muscle fibers, and increases total fiber number. In a recent study, rats were supplemented with creatine for four weeks, and their muscles were then analyzed for satellite cell activity. The investigators found a significant increase in satellite cell activity, above that normally induced by exercise alone (Dangott, Schultz, and Mozdziak 2000). Figure 12.1 illustrates how creatine may improve performance for the strength and power athlete.

The Evidence: Pro or Con?

In the first performance-related study using creatine, Dr. Greenhaff and colleagues (1993) demonstrated an improvement in muscle force during repeated bouts of isokinetic work with creatine supplementation. These responses were attributed to an increased capacity for rapid ATP replenishment from adenosine diphosphate (ADP) and PCr. This rationale is further supported by data that show that plasma ammonia levels are lower, which points to a more efficient use of adenine nucleotide stores (ATP, ADP, AMP) in the creatine group. Plasma

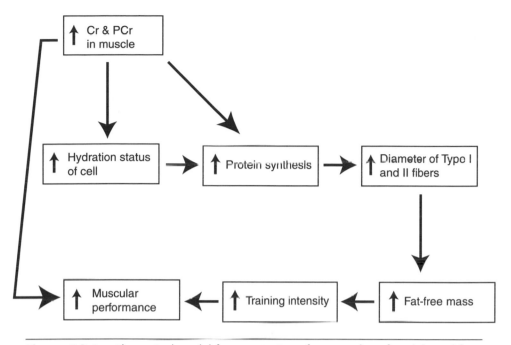

Figure 12.1 Theoretical model for creatine's performance benefits. Adpated from Volek 1996.

ammonia concentration is associated with the utilization of total adenine nucleotide stores. It is most prominent during high-intensity work efforts when adenosine monophosphate is degraded to inosine monophosphate and when adenosine is broken down to inosine. Thus, decreased plasma ammonia concentrations reflect the intracellular maintenance of ATP.

In similar studies Dr. Gaitanos and colleagues (Gaitanos et al. 1993) and Dr. Balsom and colleagues (Balsom et al. 1993) demonstrated that creatine administration could improve power output during intermittent bouts of high-intensity cycling. In subjects who performed 10 repeated six-second bouts of intense cycling interspersed with 30 seconds of rest, Dr. Gaitanos determined that the energy required to sustain mean power output during the first six-second bout was provided equally from PCr degradation and anaerobic glycolysis. These conclusions were realized from the observation that PCr stores fell by 57% while muscle lactic acid concentrations increased significantly. During the tenth sprint, however, there was no change in muscle lactate concentration while the mean power output was reduced to 73% of that generated by the first sprint. In contrast, the contribution of PCr to ATP production was calculated at nearly 80% in the final sprint and then reduced to the same extent as that of the first sprint. Because of the observed reduction in power output and contribution of anaerobic glycolysis, it was postulated that ATP regeneration was mainly derived from PCr.

To examine these observations in the accompaniment of creatine supplementation, Dr. Balsom studied subjects performing the same riding protocol as Dr. Gaitanos, using very high workloads of approximately 820 watts and 880 watts. Subjects were randomly assigned to either creatine or a placebo. The results demonstrated a decrease in blood lactic acid concentration and an accumulation of hypoxanthine at both power outputs in the creatine-supplemented group. Hypoxanthine is a blood-borne marker of adenine nucleotide breakdown during high-intensity activity; it is the intermediate step when inosine is further degraded into xanthine and uric acid (Sahlin and Katz 1993). Despite the experimental group's ability to maintain a higher performance for a longer period of time, a small yet significant decrease in aerobic power was seen in the creatine group during the 820-watt trial. Therefore, the lower levels of blood lactate concentration, coupled with lower hypoxanthine, suggest the preferential use of PCr versus ATP power generated from anaerobic glycolysis. This study also shows that creatine induced a significant increase in body mass after only six days of supplementation.

In a follow-up study, Dr. Soderlund and colleagues (Soderlund, Balsom, and Ekblom 1994) investigated whether changes in muscle metabolism occurred with creatine supplementation. They used a protocol that consisted of five six-second explosive work bouts on a cycle ergometer, combined with 30-second rest periods. After the fifth bout, an additional 10-second bout was performed as subjects tried to maintain a pedal speed of 140 rpm. Post-test trials were performed after each participant consumed 20 g creatine daily (four servings of 5 g) for six days. Results from this study revealed higher PCr concentration, lower blood lactate concentration, and a greater maintenance of intensity in 10-second work bouts in the creatine group.

In a similar study, Dr. Birch and associates (Birch, Noble, and Greenhaff 1994) used a protocol consisting of three 30-second bouts of isokinetic cycling interspersed with four minutes of rest to examine peak and mean power output, total work output, plasma ammonia concentration, and blood lactic acid concentration levels following creatine supplementation. Peak power increased by 8% in bout one while mean power output increased by 6% for bouts one and two. In contrast to similar study results, no differences were noted for blood lactic acid concentration although peak plasma ammonia concentration was lower after creatine ingestion.

Also of note is that creatine supplementation appears to help muscle PCr regeneration during recovery from maximal exercise in individuals who increase muscle creatine accumulation with supplementation (Greenhaff et al. 1994). Recent studies have demonstrated that the degree of PCr regeneration during recovery following a single bout of maximal exercise is positively related to exercise performance during a later bout of exercise (Bogdanis et al. 1998; Casey et al. 1996).

Thus, what these studies show is that creatine plays a pivotal role in the regulation and maintenance of skeletal muscle energy metabolism and fatigue. Recent data even indicate that this positive effect of creatine supplementation on strength and power performance is mediated by increasing PCr availability, primarily in fast-contracting muscle (Type II) fibers (Casey et al. 1996). We can therefore conclude that this research supports the notion that PCr depletion in fast muscle fibers limits exercise performance under these conditions (Casey et al. 1996; Hultman and Greenhaff 1991).

That conclusion certainly doesn't endorse a universal use of creatine because creatine supplementation has variable effects in those with different levels of athletic participation. Also, untrained subjects may show a greater relative increase in creatine uptake (after supplementation) compared to trained subjects (Kraemer and Volek 1999). It appears then that with well-trained athletes who have naturally higher levels of intramuscular ATP and PCr stores, supplementation has a smaller effect. Moreover, it is generally accepted that untrained athletes who participate in high-intensity, short-duration activities increase intramuscular ATP, PCr, and glycogen stores through training (MacDougall et al. 1977; Yakolev 1975). Therefore, a population that both taxes and increases its ATP and PCr stores through training may exhibit little or no response to supplementation because endogenous stores may already be at maximal levels.

In light of research data suggesting that maximal creatine accumulation is attained within three to five days after the loading phase (Harris, Soderlund, and Hultman 1992), it is of interest to explore the effects of long-term (chronic) supplementation. The first study to investigate chronic creatine use examined the effects of 28 days of creatine supplementation— 5 g taken four times daily—in resistance-trained males with 10 years experience weight lifting (Earnest et al. 1995). After 14 days of creatine use, subjects were able to perform significantly greater work on a series of three maximal anaerobic sprint bouts (stationary bicycle). After 28 days of creatine supplementation, both muscular strength and total lifting volume improved.

In a longer study, untrained, sedentary females received creatine supplements—5 g taken four times daily for four days—followed by 70 days of taking 2.5 g twice daily (Vandenberghe et al. 1997). During this latter "maintenance" period, the women underwent a resistance-training program consisting of one-hour sessions, three times weekly. After the four-day creatine-loading period, no significant improvement in arm (biceps) endurance was seen, but after 5 and 10 weeks of the low-dose creatine supplementation, arm torque was significantly greater. Similarly, measurements of strength with leg press, leg extension, and squat—one repetition maximum (1-RM)—were significantly greater in the creatine group, with fewer striking increases in bench press and leg curl and no difference in the shoulder press movement. After stopping the resistance-training program, a smaller group of subjects (seven of the original group who had received creatine) continued to take 5 g creatine daily for an additional 10 weeks. Although continued creatine usage did not prevent arm torque from declining to pretraining values, it appeared to delay the decrease in strength compared to the placebo group.

In another study, chronic creatine supplementation in NCAA Division I football players during off-season training produced significant increases in several performance variables (Kreider et al. 1998). Subjects taking a creatine mixture—5.25 g creatine taken three times daily for 28 days—displayed increases in the bench press but not for squat or power clean exercises. Muscular work performed during a series of 12 maximal cycle sprints was significantly greater during only the first five bouts with a trend for increased average total accumulated work in the creatine group. Similar results have also been noted in football players following a similar length protocol (see figure 12.2) (Stout et al. 1999).

In addition to the improvement in athletic performance—especially short-term, high-intensity activities such as weightlifting—creatine supplementation has a signficant effect on body composition. In fact, there is a plethora of data that demonstrates that creatine supplementation can augment gains in lean body mass. In one of the better studies to date, Volek et al. (1999) studied the effects of creatine supplementation—7 days at 25 g/day followed by a maintenance dose of 5 g/day for 77 days—in young experienced weight-trained males (mean age 26). Their training targeted all of the major muscle groups, three or four days per week with three or four sets of repetitions (3-12 maximum). After the 12-week training and supplementation period, the creatine-supplemented group gained an average of 9.5 lb (4.3 kg) of lean body mass compared to 4.6 lb (2.1 kg) in the placebo group. That represents a 107% difference! Another study

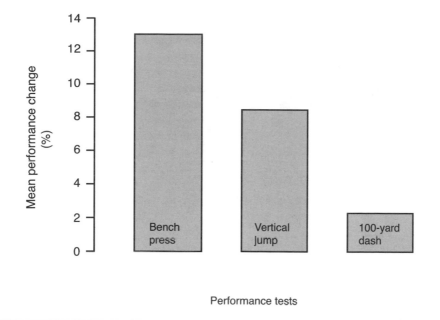

Figure 12.2 Performance change in football players. Data adapted from Stout et al. 1999.

examined creatine supplementation in NCAA Division II football players—five days at 20 g/day, followed by a maintenance dose of 0.1 or 0.3 g/kg (approximately 0.05 or 0.14 g/lb) lean body mass per day (Noonan et al. 1998). Progressive resistance training targeted all of the major muscle groups (three sets, 2-10 repetitions) four days per week plus sprint and agility training two days per week. They found that the 0.1 and 0.3 g/kg lean body mass groups gained 7.0 and 4.8 lb of lean body mass, respectively, compared with a 3.3-lb gain in the placebo. What these results illustrate is that an athlete can gain a significant amount of lean body mass with a lower dose of creatine. In other words, more isn't necessarily better. A 0.1 g/kg lean body mass dose would be equivalent to an 8 g/day dose for a 200-lb person with 15% body fat and 175 lb of lean mass.

Figure 12.3 is a compilation of several studies showing the effects of creatine supplementation on lean body mass. It is apparent that there is a range (0-10 lbs) of responses with the average response approximately being a 5-lb gain. Factors such as training status, duration of the study, sex, dosage, training program, and others affect an individual's response to creatine supplementation.

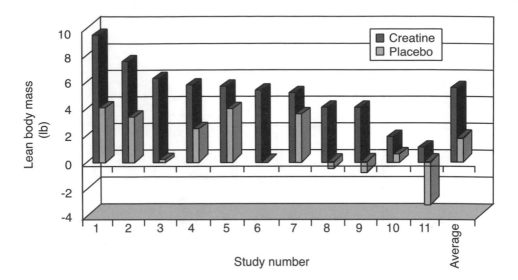

Figure 12.3 Lean body mass change after creatine supplementation. The average gain in lean body mass is approximately 5 pounds. Data adapted from Becque, Lochmann, and Melrose 2000; Earnest, Snell, Rodriguez, Almada, and Mitchell 1995; Kelly and Jenkins 1998; Kirksey, Stone, Warren et al. 1999; Kreider, Ferreira, Wilson et al. 1998; Noonan, Berg, Latin et al. 1998; Pearson, Hamby, Russel, and Harris 1999; Peeters, Lantz, and Mayhew 1999; Rawson, Wehnert, and Clarkson 1999; Vandenberghe, Goris, Van Hecke et al. 1997; and Volek, Duncan, Mazetti et al. 1999.

Guidelines for Use

Most of the studies utilized a loading phase for one week, which is 20 g per day (four doses of 5 g) for five to seven days, which should increase your skeletal muscles' creatine and PCr levels. A maintenance dose of 2.5 to 5 g per day should be enough to maintain skeletal muscle creatine and PCr levels. However, if you skip the loading phase, a dose of 3 g per day for one month will saturate your skeletal muscles. Also, the addition of carbohydrates to creatine has been shown to augment intramuscular creatine, PCr, and total creatine levels. (Green et al. 1996; Stout et al. 1999) (see table 12.2). For example, a serving of 36 g sugar (dextrose) with 5 g creatine augments performance better than creatine alone (Stout et al. 1999).

Table 12.2 Creatine Plus Carbohydrate Supplementation

	Creatine only			Creatine plus CHO*		
	Pre	Post	% change	Pre	Post	% change
PCr	85	92	+8%	84	99	+18%
Free Cr	36	50	+39%	39	57	+46%
Total Cr	122	142	+16%	123	156	+27%

Key: CHO* = carbohydrate (based on 90g of CHO added); Cr-creatine; PCr-phophocreatine; units used for measuring intramuscular levels of PCr, Free Cr, and Total Cr are mmol/kg dry muscle.

Adapted from Green et al. 1996.

Precautions

Creatine supplementation has been studied for over 10 years, and the only side effects reported have been weight gain and occasional gastrointestinal distress. There is no evidence that creatine causes cancer and no evidence that it increases the incidence of muscle cramping, heat-related illness, kidney, liver, or neural dysfunction. These are simply myths promulgated by the mainstream media. A cursory examination of the existing scientific literature clearly demonstrates that these views are grossly inaccurate.

Dehydroepiandrosterone

What Is It?

Dehydroepiandrosterone (DHEA) and its sulfate ester (DHEA-S) are steroids produced naturally by the adrenal glands and serve as precursors to both testosterone (the male sex hormone) and estrogen (female sex hormones). Interestingly, DHEA is converted in the adrenal gland into androstenedione ("andro"), which then can be converted to testosterone and estradiol. Certainly, conversion to estradiol would be an unwanted effect in athletes due to its anabolic effect on fat cells.

How Does It Work?

Like androstenedione, DHEA has been touted as a possible ergogenic aid because it can convert to testosterone. Testosterone is a potent anabolic hormone that makes it easier to accrue skeletal muscle protein. Thus, more muscle mass should translate into improved strength-power performance.

What's intriguing is that there is evidence that DHEA supplementation could "reduce the risk of heart disease, improve lipid levels, and enhance immune system function . . ." (Wallace et al. 1999). However, as it relates to athletic performance, the effect of DHEA supplementation is marginal at best.

The Evidence: Pro or Con?

In a study published in *Medicine and Science in Sports and Exercise*, scientists from LGE Performance Systems, Orlando, Florida, looked at DHEA in 40

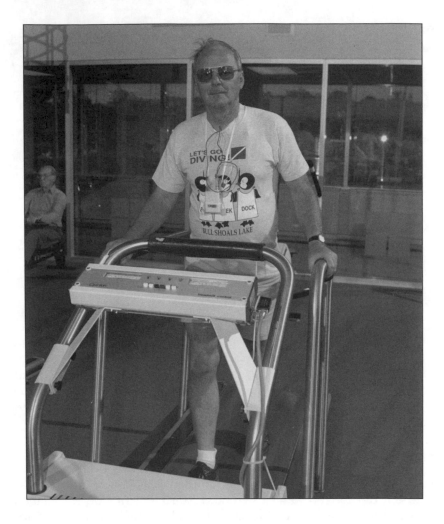

healthy, weight-trained men (average age 48) (Wallace et al. 1999). For 12 weeks, subjects consumed 100 mg DHEA daily and participated in a heavy resistance-training program. In short, researchers found no difference between the DHEA and placebo groups in the upper- and lower-body strength tests, using the bench press and leg press with one repetition maximum (1-RM). The authors did, however, state that "potential benefits would more likely be found with long-term supplementation and in special subset populations with very low initial basal levels and/or involved in high-intensity training."

Guidelines for Use

Though its ergogenic effects are questionable, a dose of 100 mg daily might offer health-related benefits. According to Yen, Morales, and Khorran (1995), DHEA in appropriate replacement doses might have remedial effects regarding immune function, muscle strength, and lean body mass; furthermore, DHEA supplementation may enhance quality of life in aging men and women with no significant adverse effects.

Precautions

In the study by Wallace et al. (1999), several subjects reported an improved sense of well-being while two subjects stated that sleep quality was adversely affected. There were no changes in plasma glucose, cholesterol, triglycerides, HDL-C, prostate-specific antigen, or liver function (ALT-transaminase). Daily DHEA supplementation at 100 mg therefore does not seem to pose a health risk, but note that DHEA is on the International Olympic Committee's list of banned substances.

Glutamine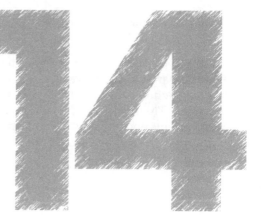

What Is It?

Glutamine is usually defined as a nonessential amino acid; you don't need to consume it to have a healthy diet. However, it should be considered a conditionally essential amino acid because during times of stress, the body's need for glutamine may not be met by the normal endogenous (within the body) synthesis of this important amino acid.

Interestingly, glutamine, not carbohydrate or fat, is the preferred fuel source for rapidly dividing cells such as enterocytes (intestinal cells) and lymphocytes (your immune system cells). Glutamine also has a role as a nitrogen carrier for acid-base balance (pH balance) and as a precursor for important macromolecules like proteins and nucleic acids. Glutamine may also have a protein-sparing effect during times of severe stress.

How Does It Work?

Glutamine is the most abundant amino acid in plasma as well as skeletal muscle; it accounts for more than 60% of the total intramuscular free amino acid pool (Lacey and Wilmore 1990; Rowbottom, Keast, and Morton 1996). In addition to skeletal muscle, adipose tissue is also a site of glutamine synthesis (Frayn et al. 1991) as are the lungs, liver, and brain. For an amino acid to be this ubiquitous, it must play important physiologic roles, and it must be quite versatile. So what exactly are the varied roles of glutamine?

First, glutamine is one of the major fuels of the gastrointestinal tract; it accounts for approximately 40% of the total glutamine that is utilized by the body. Why does the gastrointestinal tract use so much glutamine? It is due partly to the high turnover of intestinal mucosal cells and the need for continual provision of amino acids to sustain high protein synthetic rates. The health of these cells is important for the normal uptake of nutrients and as a protection against invading bacteria from the lumen of the gut. Thus, one might theorize that by providing extra exogenous glutamine via dietary supplementation, you can spare intramuscular glutamine while feeding the gastrointestinal tract—and sparing muscle glutamine is very important! Maintaining normal levels of intramuscular glutamine is important in preventing the breakdown of skeletal muscle protein (Antonio and Street 1999).

Another role of glutamine is as a fuel for cells of the immune system, kidneys, and hair follicles. Additionally, it is used in the liver for glucose and urea synthesis, and the brain utilizes glutamine as well as a precursor for neurotransmitter substances.

Therefore, it is clear that glutamine has a variety of roles in the body. Theoretically, it would make sense that by providing exogenous glutamine (i.e., supplementation), you could spare the loss of intramuscular glutamine, which would have an anti-catabolic effect. But whether extra glutamine might "boost" the immune system in normal, healthy people isn't clear at this point; however, all the evidence suggests that this amino acid is far from being "nonessential." So what is the answer? Does it help or doesn't it? Let's examine some of studies for possible conclusions.

The Evidence: Pro or Con?

Many athletes are constantly struggling with the delicate balance between building and breaking down muscle, during and after training. Perhaps the most intriguing aspect of glutamine is how it affects protein synthesis (buildup) and degradation (breakdown). The problem, though, is that nearly every study that has examined the effect of glutamine on protein balance has been done using ill patients who have undergone a severe stress, like surgery. There is at present only one study that indicates a possible anti-catabolic role of glutamine in a population of young adults who were resistance training (Candow et al. 2000).

In this study, 31 young men ingested daily either glutamine—0.4 g per lb of body weight, equivalent to 80 g for a 200-lb individual (truly a high dose!)—or a placebo (maltodextrin) for a period of six weeks. All subjects participated in a resistance training program as well. Both groups had similar increases in bench press (+14% glutamine, +13% placebo) and squat strength (+30% for both groups). Lean mass improved slightly more in the glutamine group (+2.07 lbs glutamine, +0.77 lbs placebo). In addition, they measured the rate in which muscle protein is broken down; they found that the glutamine-supplemented group had a lower rate of muscle protein degradation. According to these investigators, ". . . glutamine supplementation during resistance training has no effect on muscle performance or lean tissue mass but attenuates muscle contractile protein degradation." In simple terms, the results suggest that glutamine has a protein-sparing effect. Although there were no differences in strength or lean body mass gain, we'd suspect that if you carried the training for a longer duration, those differences may have appeared. Because glutamine seems to have protein-sparing capabilities, we can infer that it would be a good supplement to take when dieting or increasing exercise output.

An argument can also be made that glutamine might indirectly improve strength and power performance simply by keeping your immune system healthy. There's nothing worse than an illness or infection to put a major damper on your training. We all know how fast our gains can vanish when we're sick and how much hard work it takes just to return to top shape.

As stated before, glutamine is the major fuel source for lymphocytes and macrophages, the cells that fight infection and help gobble up cellular debris. Glutamine is also needed for wound repair, and there are numerous studies that show that glutamine is particularly important after a stressful or traumatic event, such as surgery. So let's now consider the recovery variable of glutamine to see if it leads us to any general conclusions about its effects.

In one study, postsurgical abdominal patients that had received glutamine—0.285 g/kg body weight per day, or 0.13 g/lb (26 g for a 200-lb person)—as part of their daily feedings had a better nitrogen balance than those that did not receive glutamine. This result was achieved by preventing the decline in protein synthesis that typically occurs following surgery. Obviously, then, in times of tremendous stress—and postsurgery is indeed stressful—glutamine is important in preventing muscle loss. But do you have to go under the knife to accrue the benefits of glutamine? Not necessarily.

In athletes who may be overtrained—and therefore slightly immunosuppressed—glutamine may be a worthwhile addition to the dietary arsenal. According to Castell and Newsholme (1998), "Oral glutamine, compared to placebo, appeared to have a beneficial effect on the incidence of infections reported by runners after a marathon." For instance, one study examined athletes who had consumed either a placebo or glutamine immediately following and two hours after running (marathon or ultramarathon) or rowing training. It was found that those athletes who consumed glutamine reported fewer infections than the placebo group (figure 14.1) (Castell, Poortmans, and Newsholme 1996). It is important to note that after training, the levels of infection were lowest in the middle-distance runners and highest in marathon (or ultramarathon) runners and in the elite rowers.

It's clear that exercise can present your body with a stress that makes it difficult for your immune system to ward off illness. Of course, weight training would probably not come close to the metabolic stress that your body endures after running 26.2 miles or farther. Perhaps the stress of rowing, which requires high power outputs as well as muscular endurance, may be more similar to the strength-power sports. Regardless, heavy training coupled with inadequate rest can contribute to a slight decline in immune system function. Giving yourself an insurance policy by ingesting glutamine may help fight off any potential infection or illness. In other words, a little glutamine supplementation may prevent you from losing training days.

Furthermore, there are other reasons that glutamine may be useful to strength-power athletes. For example, one recent study from the University of Padua in Italy found that giving glutamine with a glucose polymer promoted the storage of glycogen, particularly in the liver (Bowtell et al. 1999). In this study, seven male subjects of average physical fitness took part in three different trials. First, the subjects performed bicycle exercise designed to deplete their fast- and slow-twitch fibers of muscle glycogen. Next, they received either an 18.5% solution of glucose polymer, a dose of glutamine (8 g), or an 18.5% solution of glucose polymer plus 8 g glutamine. During the three trials, they received a continuous infusion of glucose for two hours.

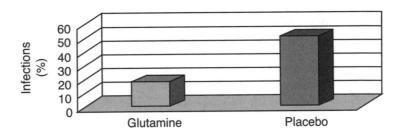

Figure 14.1 Percentage of infections in 200 runners and rowers consuming glutamine or placebo immediately or 2 hr post-exercise. Adapted from Castell et al. 1996.

Following the trials, levels of blood glutamine increased dramatically after the ingestion of glutamine alone or with the glucose polymer. In fact, glutamine concentrations were approximately 70% higher than baseline 30 to 45 minutes after glutamine ingestion. This information proves unquestionably that glutamine is not all utilized by the gastrointestinal tract. In fact, much of it is absorbed and ultimately ends up in the blood. And remember, this was only a dose of 8 g, slightly more than a teaspoon. Also note that the glutamine alone was just as effective as the glucose polymer solution in increasing muscle glycogen after the glycogen-depleting exercise bout.

So if glutamine is as effective as glucose polymer at stimulating muscle glycogen repletion, what implications does this study make regarding an athlete's diet? What it suggests is that eating a high-protein and glutamine-rich meal alone is a potent stimulator of muscle glycogen resynthesis. Add some carbohydrates and you may just have a more efficient means of storing muscle glycogen, which could significantly enhance the intensity of your workouts. Is that all we need to know? Well, not quite.

Another interesting study examines the relationship between oral glutamine consumption and growth hormone. In a study from Louisiana State University College of Medicine, researchers gave nine healthy subjects a dose of 2 g glutamine, dissolved in a cola drink (Welbourne 1995). Subjects ingested the glutamine over a 20-minute period, 45 minutes after a light breakfast. Eight of the nine subjects had a significant rise in plasma glutamine at 30 and 60 minutes. Glutamine levels then returned to normal at 90 minutes, but interestingly, plasma growth hormone levels were significantly *higher* at 90 minutes. This study suggests that even a small dose (2 g, less than half a teaspoon) can elicit an elevation in plasma growth hormone. So what exactly are the physiological implications of these results? An explanation of growth hormone is needed to more clearly illustrate the answer to this question.

Growth hormone (GH) is released from the pituitary gland in the brain; it has positive effects on virtually every tissue in the body. For example, GH promotes the utilization of stored body fat as an energy source. Additionally, GH causes indirect activation of other hormones, such as insulin-like growth factor 1 (IGF-1), which promotes protein synthesis for building muscle and connective tissue. Furthermore, this stimulation speeds up repair processes and recovery from exercise and illness. By having a direct effect on new bone formation and by increasing availability and absorption of calcium and phosphate, GH may largely reduce the effects of osteoporosis caused by menopause and aging.

Having established this definition of GH, we can now consider how it may affect the strength-power athlete. Theoretically, glutamine—via changes in GH—helps promote muscle mass gain and perhaps fat loss; thus, this theory translates into larger muscles. Larger muscles then translate into better strength or power.

Guidelines for Use

A minimum of 2 g glutamine is needed to elicit an increase in plasma growth hormone levels, and 8 g glutamine is effective in promoting glycogen resynthesis. Doses as high as 80 g (for a 200-lb person) seem to indicate an anti-catabolic effect in those who exercise. Certainly, 80 g glutamine is probably not feasible for athletes interested in using this amino acid. It should be recognized that doses needed to favorably alter protein balance (from the studies done in hospital patients) are fairly substantial—0.2 to 0.6 g per kg body weight. At the lower end, that would translate to approximately 0.1 g per lb of bodyweight, or 20 g for a 200-lb person. In other words, an effective working dose could potentially be 10% of one's body weight.

It should also be recognized that glutamine supplementation need not be cycled; that is, one should not alternate between off and on periods of use. Because glutamine may be intimately involved in the recovery process, the consumption of it as part of a postexercise meal is important.

Precautions

Studies from Ziegler et al. (1990) have shown that short- and long-term glutamine supplementation is safe in humans. Oral doses of glutamine—0.1-0.3 g/kg body weight, or approximately 0.05-0.13 g/lb—produce an acute rise in plasma glutamine as well as in amino acids known to be end products of glutamine metabolism (i.e., alanine, citrulline, arginine). However, there was no evidence of toxicity as demonstrated by no change in ammonia or glutamate levels. Based on data derived from glutamine feeding as part of total parenteral nutrition, a dose in the range of 0.285 to 0.570 g/kg body weight (or 0.13-0.26 g/lb body weight; 26-52 g for a 200-lb person) would seem safe. However, such a large dose may not be feasible for most individuals. We would speculate that 25-50% of that dose may be helpful for the strength-power athlete.

Ipriflavone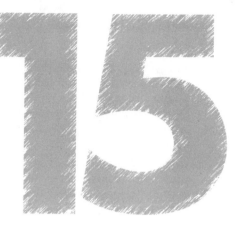

What Is It?

Ipriflavone is a derivative from phytoestrogen, a chemical found in plants that have weak estrogenic activity. A type of phytoestrogen is the isoflavone (Kuiper et al. 1998), and there are a variety of isoflavones that might have potential effects on body composition. These include ipriflavone and also methoxyisoflavone (5-methyl-7-methoxyisoflavone).

How Does It Work?

Ipriflavone is one of the most commonly studied isoflavones and is a synthetic phytoestrogen made from the soy isoflavone daidzein. There is actually quite an abundance of evidence that ipriflavone has anabolic effects in bone (Gennari et al. 1998). According to the *Alternative Medicine Review*, "Preliminary studies have also found ipriflavone effective in preventing bone loss associated with steroid use, immobility, ovariectomy, renal osteodystrophy, and gonadotropin hormone-releasing hormone agonists". The way ipriflavone works is by inhibiting bone resorption (removal).

One commercially available isoflavone is 5-methyl-7-methoxy-isoflavone, and preliminary evidence (discussed in next section) suggests a possible effect on human body composition. It isn't known why this might occur, though.

The Evidence: Pro or Con?

To date, there have been no studies on healthy, resistance-trained humans on the effects of ipriflavone, but what is interesting is that over 60 clinical studies have been performed on ipriflavone as an antiosteoporosis agent. One study, published in *Calcified Tissue International* (Agnusdei et al. 1997a), compared the effects of ipriflavone (200 mg, three times per day) with a placebo over a two-year study using postmenopausal women (aged 50-65 years). Each subject received a daily supplement of calcium (1 g). At one year, the ipriflavone-supplemented group experienced a 1.4% increase in vertebral bone density and a 1% increase after the two-year period. The placebo group had a significant drop in bone density.

The gain in bone mass also represents a gain in lean body mass; however, to get an improvement in indices of strength or power, one would need to additionally seek a gain in skeletal muscle mass. Unfortunately, there is no evidence at this time that ipriflavone has such an effect, but let's examine one more type of isoflavone to see if we can draw any general conclusions.

Although data is limited, the isoflavone 5-methyl-7-methoxyisoflavone ("methoxy") has been examined and researched as a potential ergogenic aid. In a study from the University of Nebraska (Antonio, Incledon, and Van Gammeren 2000), 14 healthy, resistance-trained men (average age 21-22) consumed either a placebo or 800 mg methoxy daily for eight weeks. Each subject participated in the same heavy resistance-training program. Bone-free lean body mass and percentage body fat improved more in the methoxy group than in the placebo group (figure 15.1).

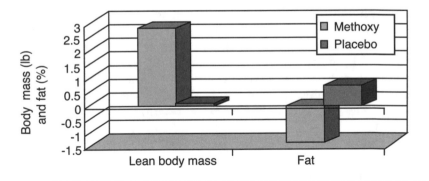

Figure 15.1 Average change in lean body mass and percentage fat. Adapted from Antonio et al. 2000.

According to the United States patent #4,163,746, there are other isoflavones that are "particularly active as anabolic agents" (Feuer et al. 1979). These include 5-methyl-7-methoxy-isoflavone, 5-methyl-7-ethoxy-isoflavone, 5-methyl-7-(2-hydroxy-ethoxy)-isoflavone, and 5-methyl-7-isopropoxy-isoflavone. Future studies need to verify whether these compounds genuinely have anabolic effects.

Guidelines for Use

The limited information suggests that a daily dose of 800 mg 5-methyl-7-methoxyisoflavone may have positive effects on body composition; however, further research is needed to verify this. It is clear that ipriflavone can enhance bone mineral content in older women, but whether this translates to a similar effect in young healthy men or women is questionable. It is our contention that there is not enough evidence to support the use of ipriflavones as an aid to promote skeletal muscle hypertrophy.

Precautions

Although uncommon, gastrointestinal problems may occur in those taking ipriflavone (Agnusdei et al. 1997b). There are no reported side effects of the 5-methyl-7-methoxyisoflavone.

Norandrostenedione and Norandrostenediol

What Are They?

Collectively called norsteroids, norandrostenedione (nordione) and norandrostenediol (nordiol) are steroids that are similar in structure to androstenedione and androstenediol, respectively. The difference is that the 19th carbon of androstenedione and androstenediol is removed. It has been suggested that androstenedione exerts its anabolic effects via its conversion to testosterone; however, this mechanism does not apply to the norsteroids. Instead, it is thought that the norsteroids bind directly to the androgen receptor and promote increases in protein synthesis, thus resulting in larger muscles.

How Do They Work?

Because the norsteroids are thought to bind to the androgen receptor, we can confer a muscle-building or anabolic effect with the androgen receptor (AR) being found in the skeletal muscle. For instance, whenever testosterone, the primary male sex hormone, binds to the AR, it sets into play a series of biochemical events that ultimately result in an increase in muscle protein and thus bigger muscles. Can we then conclude that the norsteroids, specifically nordione and nordiol, have a similar effect? Let's examine the evidence.

The Evidence: Pro or Con?

Though several studies have examined the safety and efficacy of androstenedione ("andro"), there is a dearth of information on the norsteroids. In fact, there is only one peer-reviewed study on the norsteroids. A study from the University of Nebraska-Kearney (Van Gammeren, Falk, and Antonio 2001) examined the effects of eight weeks of norsteroid supplementation on body composition and athletic performance in weight-trained males. These recreational bodybuilders received either a combination of 100 mg 19-nor-4-androstene-3,17-dione (N-dione) and 56 mg 19-nor-4-androstene-3,17-diol (N-diol) (156 mg total norsteroid per day) or a vitamin placebo for an eight-week duration. In addition, they each participated in a bodybuilding training program four days a week. From this limited study, it was found that low-dose supplementation with norsteroids has no effect on body composition or exercise performance in resistance-trained young men (see figures 16.1 and 16.2). Even though the norsteroids group experienced a relatively greater gain in bench press strength, this difference was not statistically significant. Perhaps a larger sample size may show norsteroids to be effective.

Guidelines for Use

As of now, there isn't much data on the norsteroids. Though the study by Van Gammeren et al. (2001) showed no effects, it should be noted that the dosage was quite low. A higher dose may be needed to induce an anabolic

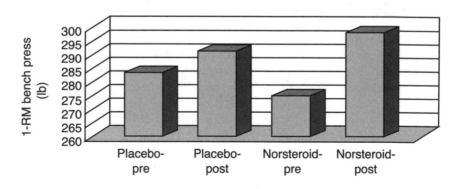

Figure 16.1 Bench press, one repetition maximum (1-RM) before and after 8-week study. Adapted from Van Gammeren et al. 2001.

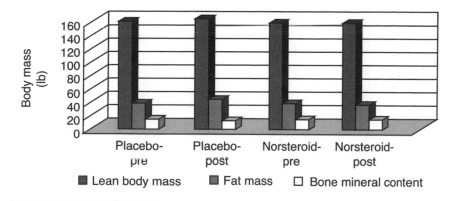

Figure 16.2 Change in lean body mass, fat mass, and bone mineral content in norsteroids study. Adapted from Van Gammeren et al. 2001.

effect. Perhaps a dose of 0.5-1.0 g daily for a two-month cycle with a similar length off-cycle might have an ergogenic effect. Certainly, future studies are needed to clarify the effects of the norsteroids.

Precautions

There have been no safety studies on these particular norsteroids although the few existing studies have not reported any harmful effects. Regardless, norandrostenedione and norandrostenediol are on the International Olympic Committee's banned substance list.

It is important to note that for those who compete at the elite level and abide by the rules of the various governing bodies (NCAA, IOC), the use of the general, over-the-counter norsteroids may elicit a positive drug test. For example, you can test positive for nandrolone if you ingest norsteroids (Uralets and Gillette 1999). Also, in a study published in the *Journal of Strength and Conditioning Research*, scientists (Colker et al. 2001) evaluated the short-term effects of norsteroid ingestion (norandrostenedione and norandrostenediol). Subjects ingested the steroids at two doses, 72 mg or 144 mg, daily for 10 days. All subjects tested positive for nortestosterone, an illicit anabolic steroid, on days 3, 5, 7, and 10. Interestingly, there wasn't a change in the urinary testosterone:epitestosterone ratio on any day, and at least in the short-term, there were no changes in liver or kidney function. Bottom line: If you're a competitive athlete, the ingestion of these steroids may in fact produce a positive drug test.

Octacosanol

17

What Is It?

Octacosanol is a waxy substance found in wheat germ oil (Bucci 1993) and sugar cane. Chemically, it is a long-chain (C_{28}) waxy alchohol (Wolinksy 1998).

How Does It Work?

Octacosanol is not known to have any anabolic or anti-catabolic effects on muscle tissue itself; however, it may play a role in muscle and strength development by acting on nerve tissue because one aspect of increasing strength is via neural adaptation (Kraemer et al. 1996). Theoretically, if athletes supplement to make the nervous system act more efficiently, it may facilitate speed and strength production as well as influence the growth response in skeletal muscle by activating more muscle fibers during a given lift.

The Evidence: Pro or Con?

Limited research suggests that octacosanol supplementation may have ergogenic properties in activities requiring a high degree of quickness (reaction time). Specific instances that may be aided by octacosanol include the following: Squatting and pressing in explosive sports like power lifting and Olympic weightlifting; getting out of the blocks quickly in a sprint race; getting off the line quickly after the snap in football; and rapid throwing movements in baseball.

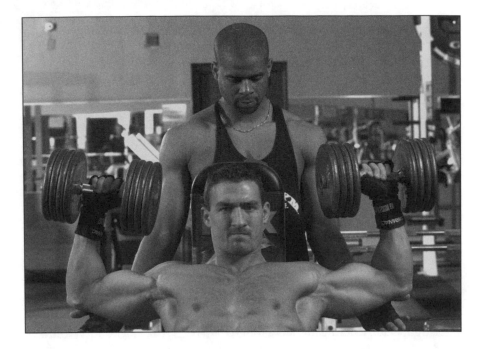

The study most commonly referenced that demonstrates performance-enhancing benefits of octacosanol was conducted using 1 mg/day, given for eight weeks (Saint-John and McNaughton 1986). The supplement was administered in a double-blind fashion using 16 subjects. Results showed that those receiving octacosanol had improved reaction time to visual stimuli as well as a significant increase in grip strength. There were no differences in endurance time as measured by cycle ergometry.

Guidelines for Use

The limited data suggests that 1 mg octacosanol per day may improve reaction time, but to date, there have been no replicative studies to support this finding. The use of octocosanol deserves further investigation to conclusively support this claim.

Precautions

This substance has been widely used as a food and nutritional supplement since the 1950s, and there are no reports in the literature reporting toxicity in animals or humans. Its use by athletes is not common, though. Thus, it isn't known if harmful effects might occur from long-term use or from higher dose consumption.

Ornithine Alpha-Ketoglutarate

18

What Is It?

Ornithine alpha-ketoglutarate (OKG) is formed from two molecules of the amino acid ornithine and one molecule of alpha-ketoglutarate (a metabolite of the Krebs cycle). OKG is marketed as an anti-catabolic agent that helps reduce muscle protein breakdown.

How Does It Work?

OKG has been shown in a variety of studies to have an anabolic or anti-catabolic effect. Most of the studies on OKG that show positive results have been on patients suffering from burns, malnutrition, or postsurgery. How OKG exerts these effects isn't known, but the secretion of hormones such as insulin and growth hormone—as well as its conversion to other metabolites like glutamine and arginine—might play a role.

The Evidence: Pro or Con?

Similar to glutamine, OKG might have a protein-sparing effect, particularly during what is called a "hypercatabolic state." A hypercatabolic state exists during times of severe physical stress, such as after suffering a burn, postsurgery, or prolonged illness. Some scientists theorize that this could also apply to intense exercise training or better yet, overtraining. Vanbourdolle et al. (1987) showed that the enteral (via the intestine) administration of OKG to burn patients improved glucose tolerance. Varying doses of OKG (10, 20, and 30 g) delivered as a bolus or via continuous infusion were found to improve nitrogen balance; furthermore, urinary 3-methylhistidine was reduced (an indicator of muscle protein degradation) (De Bandt et al. 1998). The administration of 30 g as a bolus seemed to have the greatest benefit. Of course, 30 g is quite a large dose and may make the consumption of OKG unfeasible.

But let's examine whether or not OKG actually helps strength-power athletes. In a recently published study, researchers examined the effects of OKG on healthy, weight-trained men (Chetlin et al. 2000). Eighteen resistance-trained men (aged 18-35) took part in a double-blind, placebo-controlled, six-week study. They were randomly assigned to either a placebo group or a OKG-supplemented group (dose of 10 g/day as capsules). They did a variety of exercise and blood tests. OKG had no effect on glucose, insulin, or growth hormone levels nor did it have any effect on resting heart rate or blood pressure. Interestingly, changes in squat strength did not differ between groups, yet the OKG-supplemented group had a greater relative increase in bench press strength (figure 18.1).

At least from this one study, it's apparent that OKG doesn't have an effect on the anabolic hormones insulin and growth hormone. In fact, other clinical work has shown that OKG administered to burn patients had no effect on plasma insulin or growth hormone concentration (Vanbourdolle et al. 1987).

This isn't to say that OKG doesn't produce effects, though. For instance, in growth-retarded, prepubertal children, 15 g OKG produced an increase in plasma insulin-like growth factor-1 (Moukarzel et al. 1994). Also, why the subjects in the Chetlin et al. study (previously mentioned) experienced an improvement in upper-body strength but not in the lower body is

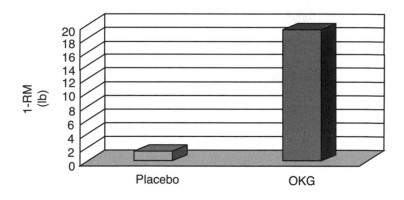

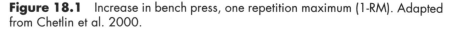

Figure 18.1 Increase in bench press, one repetition maximum (1-RM). Adapted from Chetlin et al. 2000.

inexplicable. Because no change was seen in muscle mass in either group, perhaps the changes in strength seen in the OKG-supplemented group were mediated by changes in the central nervous system. Either way, the use of OKG as an ergogenic aid is ripe for future research.

Guidelines for Use

From the single study that demonstrated an improvement in bench press strength, a daily 10 g dose for at least six weeks might elicit an ergogenic effect. It isn't known if lower doses for longer durations elicit similar effects; conversely, the effects of higher doses in healthy, weight-trained athletes need further examination as well.

Precautions

High-dose OKG administration (up to 30 g/day) in humans has not been shown to have harmful side effects. Short-term (six weeks), relatively high-dose OKG (10 g/day) consumption has also not been shown to be harmful.

Protein

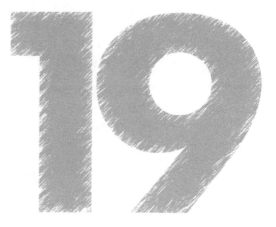

What Is It?

Not only does protein serve a multitude of roles in the human body, but there are also many types of protein that the body uses: contractile protein in skeletal muscle; cytoskeletal (structural) proteins in skeletal muscle; enzymes, as components of cells and cell membranes; and hormones. Proteins, however, are not classically considered fuel sources, like fat and carbohydrates. For instance, adipose tissue (fat cells) is only 15% water whereas muscle is 80% water and 20% protein (not all of it contractile).

What serves as the building blocks of protein are the amino acids. Although the primary function of protein—as it relates to strength-power sports—is to provide these needed amino acids for maintaining an anabolic state (a growth state), there are times when protein may actually be used as a fuel source. This phenomenon usually occurs when you're in a carbohydrate-depleted state, like when you are on a low-carbohydrate diet or are exercising continuously for over two hours. What most athletes want, though, is to maintain the absolute highest levels of anabolism (muscle building) possible. Because one of the components of proteins is the molecule nitrogen (16% of protein), scientists measure this anabolic level through nitrogen balance. When you eat protein, you're taking in, among other things, nitrogen; therefore, if you want to put muscle on, you want to take in more nitrogen (protein) than you're breaking down. A positive nitrogen balance exists when protein intake exceeds protein degradation. The opposite of that, a negative nitrogen balance, exists when you don't consume enough protein; that is, more nitrogen is excreted than consumed in your diet.

How Does It Work?

The recommended daily allowance (RDA) of 0.8 g protein per kg body weight (approximately 0.4 g/lb, or 80 g for a 200-lb person) is too low for athletes. Although muscle protein breakdown increases during exercise, there is a significant increase in muscle protein synthesis for at least 24 hours after resistance or aerobic exercise. Current research suggests that 1.5 to 2.0 g per kg body weight per day (0.7-0.9 g/lb, or 140-180 g/day for a 200-lb person) is actually what is needed for those interested in packing on some muscle (Lemon et al. 1997). Anecdotally, many athletes, particularly bodybuilders, consume as much as 1 g protein per lb body weight (see table 19.1). The need for extra dietary protein is based on the notion that extra amino acids are needed to repair injured muscle fibers and to promote gains in muscle mass.

The Evidence: Pro or Con?

According to Rennie and Tipton (2000), "There is no evidence that habitual exercise increases protein requirements; indeed protein metabolism may become more efficient as a result of training." Furthermore, Wolfe (2000) states "it is not possible to form a consensus position regarding the benefit of protein or amino acid supplements in exercise training." Disagreement among scientists is common and accepted within the scientific community, but athletes can't wait for scientists to come to a consensus to determine if they should increase their protein intake above the RDA.

We could all wait for apples to levitate tomorrow, yet we won't rewrite Newton's laws in anticipation of it. Hence, the practice of consuming protein in excess of the RDA is quite common among strength-power

Table 19.1 Protein/Energy Needs in Strength-Power Versus Endurance Athletes

	Strength-power athlete	Endurance athlete
Body weight (kg)	100.0	60.0
Recommended grams of protein/kg body weight	1.8	1.4
Total protein, grams/day	180.0	84.0
Kcals/kg body weight	44.0	44.0
Total kcals/day	4,400.0	2,640.0

Adapted from Williams 1998.

athletes, and this practice is almost synonymous with strength-power athletes. So either they're completely misguided and wasting their time and money, or there may actually be a benefit to consuming large quantities of protein. One would at least admit that if the practice had no utility, it would have faded with other snake-oil supplements such as boron, ground up bull's testes, and ferulic acid. For the time being, let's examine perhaps why extra protein consumption may be helpful.

After a bout of resistance exercises, muscle protein synthesis is elevated for 24 to 48 hours (MacDougall et al. 1995; Tipton and Wolfe 2001). It would make sense then that to increase total muscle mass, it would be necessary to provide exogenous amino acids. Ultimately, there has to be a net accretion of muscle protein because this added protein has to be acquired from somewhere (i.e., from an athlete's diet). According to Tarnopolsky et al. (1992), strength-power athletes need to consume approximately 1.76 g protein daily per kg body weight (0.8 g/lb, or 160 g for a 200-lb person). This recommendation is more than twice the requirement for inactive, sedentary individuals. To be on the so-called safe side, many athletes consume more than this amount, and popular magazines even suggest that bodybuilders consume 1 g of protein per lb body weight (i.e., 2.2 g of protein per kg body weight). Your math is correct; that's a whopping 200 g for a 200-lb person—over twice the RDA for an inactive individual.

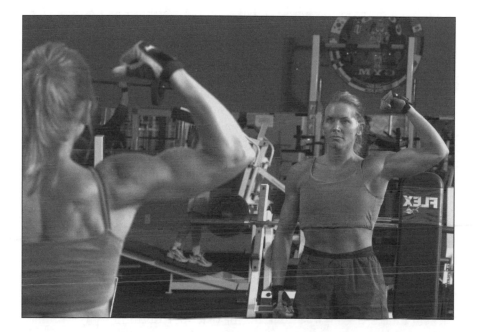

Why would an athlete need this extra protein? Two reasons: First is to repair muscle fibers that have been damaged as a result of exercise, and second is to provide the extra amino acids needed to promote skeletal muscle hypertrophy. Studies by Peter Lemon, PhD, verified the need for increased dietary protein requirements in active individuals (Lemon et al. 1997; Lemon 1998, 2000).

Guidelines for Use

Consuming protein in excess of the RDA is certainly not harmful to healthy athletes (see "Precautions"). Thus, it would behoove strength-power athletes to consume *at least* 1.5 g protein per kg body weight daily (approximately 0.7 g/lb, or 140 g for a 200-lb person). The best sources of protein include beef, chicken, fish, pork, and an assortment of meal replacement powders that contain various combinations of whey, casein, or soy protein.

Precautions

Poortmans and Dellalieux (2000) studied the effects of high and medium protein intake in bodybuilders and other well-trained athletes. Subjects underwent blood and urine sampling and kept a seven-day food record. Despite higher plasma concentrations of uric acid and calcium, the group of bodybuilders on the high-protein diet had normal renal clearance of creatine, urea, and albumin. Interestingly, the nitrogen balance for both groups became positive when daily protein intake exceeded 1.26 g per kg body weight (approximately 0.6 g/lb). According to these scientists, "It appears that protein intake under 2.8 g/kg/day [1.3 g/lb/day] does not impair renal function in well-trained athletes as indicated by the measures of renal function used in this study." To paraphrase, there is no evidence that in normal, healthy individuals, consuming large quantities of dietary protein is harmful. In an intriguing animal study, Zaragoza et al. (1987) fed rats a diet of 80% protein for more than half of their life span, and they found no harmful effects of this very high intake of protein.

Other purported health risks include an increased rate of calcium excretion due to high-protein consumption. This means that if you eat too much protein, you lose bone mass and set yourself up for osteoporosis down the road, right? Wrong. According to a study published in the *Journal of Bone Mineral Research* (Hannan et al. 2000), "Lower protein intake was significantly related to bone loss at the femoral (hip) and spine bone mineral density sites." They go on to state that "higher intake of animal protein does not appear to affect the skeleton adversely . . ." Therefore, increased protein intake does not set one up for osteoporosis, and a high-protein diet for athletes does not seem to have any damaging effects.

Ribose

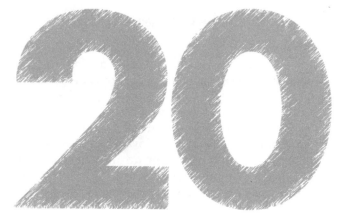

What Is It?

D-ribose (ribose) is a natural simple sugar found in every cell of the body. Ribose is used to make energy for muscles, heart, and other tissues and may be important when a person is very active. Ribose looks and tastes like powdered sugar.

How Does It Work?

Ribose is immediately absorbed into the body's cells and converted to useful energy. Cells can make ribose from sugar, but the problem is that this process is slow. When the energy demand is not great, alternative carbohydrates work fine. But during intense activity, energy is used up faster than it can be replenished, and muscles therefore become fatigued. This imbalance is why athletes feel tired and sore after an intense exercise session. Taking supplemental ribose so that it is available during and after a workout gives muscles a source of "high octane" fuel that is readily available; it speeds the process of recovering energy molecules and lessens fatigue and soreness (Burke 1999).

Ribose also forms part of the backbone of the main energy molecule for the cell, adenosine triphosphate (ATP). When muscles need energy, the ATP molecule splits up, giving off bursts of energy with each split. Ribose is therefore needed for two reasons: one, because it is part of ATP and two, because it enhances the reactions that lead to rebuilding ATP for the next required bursts of energy (Burke 1999).

As you work out, especially during intense workouts under anaerobic conditions such as sprints or bouts of resistance exercise, your ATP breaks up into its fundamental building blocks and is slow to be recovered. If these building blocks are not captured and rebuilt into ATP, they are washed from the cell and lost into the bloodstream. The process of making new building blocks is very slow, which is why it can take two to three days (or more) to recover after an intense workout or competition. Ribose supplementation speeds the recovery of these energy-building blocks and provides immediate fuel for the following exercise session and the speedier recovery (Burke 1999).

The Evidence: Pro or Con?

Knowledge about the effect of ribose in the heart has been gathered over the past 25 years in many laboratory and clinical studies in both humans and animals (Pauli and Pepine 2000). These studies have shown many positive effects of ribose, including improved heart function and enhanced recovery of ATP in the heart after decreased blood flow or during exercise on a treadmill. More recent studies on the benefits of ribose for athletes developed out of the rationale that during intense exercise, similar energy limitations were occurring in other muscles beyond those of the heart.

In one of these studies, 16 college-aged men participated in intense exercise bouts on a stationary cycle twice a day (Witter et al. 2000; Gallagher et al. 2000c). In this study, the participants took a dose of either glucose placebo or 10 g ribose, two times per day. The results showed that those subjects taking supplemental ribose had a larger increase in mean power over five days of training (4.2% vs. 0.6%) and greater peak power output at the last sprint session than the group taking glucose (11.4 watts/kg vs. 10.4 watts/kg, or 5.2 watts/lb vs. 4.7 watts/lb). Throughout the entire training sessions, the mean power output was consistently higher in the subjects who took ribose than in the subjects who took the glucose placebo. Fatigue was also consistently less in the ribose group than in the placebo group.

In another study, exercise performance was measured in male bodybuilders for over four weeks (Antonio, Falk, and Van Gammeren 2001). The subjects were randomly divided into two groups, with 10 subjects in each group. The supplements were taken in divided doses: 5 g taken 15 minutes before the workout and another 5 g immediately following it, for a total of 10 g per day. The ribose group experienced a significant increase in the number of bench press repetitions performed for 10 sets to muscular failure (+19.6% ribose vs. +12.0% placebo) and a significant increase in maximal strength.

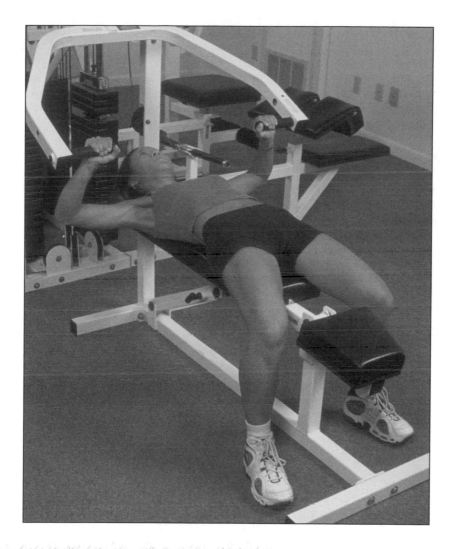

Guidelines for Use

The use of ribose deserves consideration though some of it is speculative. Ribose is most useful when taken around the time of exercise. It can be taken before, during, or right after a workout. The greatest benefit is experienced when ribose is available to the muscle as it needs it, which is when much of the muscle energy stores are being used up. For a casual exerciser, this point may not happen until toward the end of a workout. For the serious athlete who has longer workouts, ribose may be needed midway through an exercise session. The best way to be sure to optimize the effect of ribose is to split the dose so that some is available during the workout and some immediately afterward during recovery (Burke 1999).

Recommended doses seem to be from 1 to 10 g, with higher doses appearing more likely to result in greater benefit. For those who want to maximize the potential benefits should take 5 g before and 5 g after each exercise session.

Precautions

Taking high doses of ribose (10 g or more) on an empty stomach may lead to temporary light-headedness. It is recommended that single doses should be 5 g or less unless they are taken with sports drinks, juice, or food.

Sodium Bicarbonate

21

What Is It?

Sodium bicarbonate (SB) is an antacid (alkalinizing agent), meaning that it counteracts acid. Sodium bicarbonate is naturally formed in the body and is also found in baking soda.

How Does It Work?

During high-intensity exercise, production of adenosine triphosphate (ATP) from anaerobic glycolysis produces lactic acid. Lactic acid decreases the pH in the muscle cells, and a low pH may interfere with the muscle contraction process and with energy production. Once the SB is ingested and gets into the bloodstream, however, the pH in the blood increases. The pH difference created between the inside and outside of muscle cells induces an accelerated movement of H+ ions; they move out of the working muscle tissue and into the extracellular spaces, which consequently raises the intracellular (inside the muscle cell) pH (Ibanez et al. 1995). This intracellular increase reduces the negative effects of lactic acid (low pH) and thus allows athletes to perform high-intensity exercise longer before the onset of fatigue.

The Evidence: Pro or Con?

Many researchers have investigated the effects of sodium bicarbonate on strength and power performance. While some studies show no significant increase, a majority seem to indicate that SB increases maximal exercise performance. McNaughton and colleagues (1999) conducted a five-day study that investigated the effects of ingesting SB before a short-term, high-intensity cycling exercise. Before the workout, males ingested 500 mg SB per kg body weight (approximately 227 mg/lb, or about 45 g in a 200-lb person). The results showed that ingestion of sodium bicarbonate over a period of five days significantly improved total work capacity and power by 12% and 10%, respectively. In a similar study done earlier, McNaughton and colleagues (1997) investigated the effects of sodium bicarbonate on high-intensity cycling exercise in moderately trained

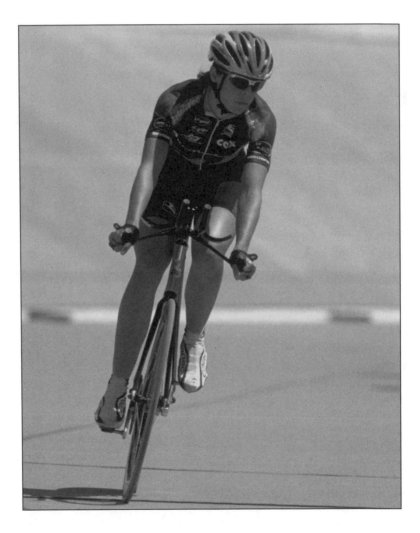

women. The results also demonstrated a significant increase in total work capacity (9%) and peak power (9%).

In addition to the studies that examined the effects of SB on high-intensity workouts, Drs. Coombes and McNaughton (1993) investigated whether a similar oral dose of SB would improve isokinetic strength and endurance: "The results indicate there was a significant increase in both the amount of work completed—isokinetic endurance—and the peak torque or isokinetic strength . . ." The findings in all of these studies are in agreement with several other studies that support the claim that SB supplementation enhances strength and power performance (Linderman and Gosselink 1994; Matson and Tran 1993: McNaughton 1992a, 1992b; McNaughton et al. 1991, 1997, 1999; Vebitsky et al. 1997).

Guidelines for Use

Despite the fact that many studies favor sodium bicarbonate as an effective supplement, there are several factors that must be considered. First, the dosages in those studies, as well as most other studies showing positive results, are quantities of 300 to 500 mg per kg body weight or greater (approximately 136-227 mg/lb, or about 27-45 g for a 200-lb person). Such dosages have been associated with side effects such as diarrhea, cramping, nausea, and vomiting. These side effects are reduced when using doses of 100 to 200 mg per kg body weight (about 45-90 mg/lb, or 9-18 g for a 200-lb person).

The problem, however, is that these smaller doses seem to be ineffective at improving strength and power performance. Linderman and colleagues (1992) investigated the efficacy of using smaller doses of sodium bicarbonate. The researchers examined the effects of 200 mg sodium bicarbonate per kg body weight (about 90 mg/lb, or 18 g for a 200-lb person) rather than higher dosages commonly used on a short-term, maximal exercise capacity. Dr. Linderman and colleagues reported that this dosage, given before the workout, did not improve performance. In agreement, several other studies suggest that oral administration of sodium bicarbonate may not be effective at doses less than or equal to 300 mg per kg body weight (about 136 mg/lb, or 27 g for a 200-lb person) (Gaitanos et al. 1991; Horswill et al. 1988; Tiryaki and Atterbom 1995; Webster et al. 1993). Additionally, the time when the sodium bicarbonate is ingested can affect its ability to influence performance. Most studies had subjects ingest sodium bicarbonate 90 minutes prior to exercise, which allowed the concentration of SB in the blood to increase, thus making it a more effective buffer.

Precautions

Side effects associated with sodium bicarbonate supplementation at doses of 300 mg per kg (136 mg/lb) body weight or higher are fairly severe, causing problems such as diarrhea, cramping, nausea, and vomiting. These side effects have been reduced when subjects drink an abundance of water or when lower doses are used. It is always best to try this supplement first during a practice session before using it as a precompetition aid.

Sodium Citrate

What Is It?

Citrate is basically a sodium molecule attached to a metabolic intermediate. In other words, it is a Krebs cycle intermediate, and it can be found in common foods such as citrus fruits. This combination of sodium with a metabolic intermediate may affect your blood's pH in such a manner that it may help athletic performance.

How Does It Work?

Although sodium citrate is not actually a base, it can increase blood pH without the gastrointestinal distress that is caused by sodium bicarbonate (Van Someren et al. 1998). It is believed that once in the blood, sodium citrate actually breaks down into bicarbonate and thus ultimately increases the extracellular pH (Tiryaki and Atterbom 1995). If this is truly the case, sodium citrate would provide a means as a supplement to arbitrarily raise extracellular pH and, consequently, maintain a neutral environment that is necessary for an athlete's performance.

This transformation is made possible through the mechanism that lies in the increased pH created between the muscle and blood (Cox and Jenkins 1994). During high-intensity exercise, anaerobic glycolysis continually produces H+ ions, which decrease the pH in the muscle cells. Once the sodium citrate gets into the bloodstream after oral ingestion, the pH in the blood then increases. It is this pH difference that induces an accelerated movement of H+ ions out of the working muscle tissue and into the extracellular spaces. This movement consequently raises the intracellular pH to the degree needed to reduce the negative effects of lactic acid (low pH) (Ibanez et al. 1995). Thus, using sodium citrate to balance the pH allows athletes to perform longer before the onset of fatigue.

The Evidence: Pro or Con?

The research concerning sodium citrate's performance-enhancing effects for the strength-power athlete seem to be equivocal at best. In fact, most of the studies illustrate sodium citrate as having no ergogenic effects on short duration, high-intensity exercise (Ball and Maughan 1997; Cox and Jenkins 1994; Kowalchuk et al. 1989; Parry-Billings and MacLaren 1986; Van Someren et al. 1998). Because short-term, high-intensity activities— those lasting less than 60 seconds—do not allow lactic acid production to reach a maximum, sodium citrate's buffering capabilities are not fully utilized; thus, a sodium citrate supplement wouldn't be effective in this context (Parry-Billings and MacLaren 1986). In exercise lasting between 2 and 15 minutes, however, sodium citrate has been shown to have a higher success rate in improving exercise performance. It needs to be taken 90 minutes before high-intensity exercise in doses of 0.5 g per kg body weight (about 0.2 g/lb, or 40 g for a 200-lb person) (Linossier et al. 1997; McNaughton and Cedaro 1992). Furthermore, Hausswirth and colleagues (1995) reported a significant improvement (about 20% greater) in leg endurance when subjects were supplemented before maximal isometric knee extension with a lower dose of sodium citrate, 0.4 g per kg body weight (a little less than 0.2 g/lb).

Guidelines for Use

Given 60 to 90 minutes before high-intensity events (those lasting for more than 2 minutes and up to 15 minutes), a single dose of 0.4 to 0.5 g sodium citrate per kg of body mass (36-40 g for a 200 lb person) may see the greatest benefit of supplementation. Before using with any major sporting event, the dose and timing of sodium citrate supplementation should be well tested to ensure tolerability and effectiveness.

Precautions

One of the advantages sodium citrate may have over other buffers (like sodium bicarbonate) is that it is well tolerated by most users; very few subjects have reported gastrointestinal distress during the use of sodium citrate (McNaughton 1990). It should not be overlooked that nausea was

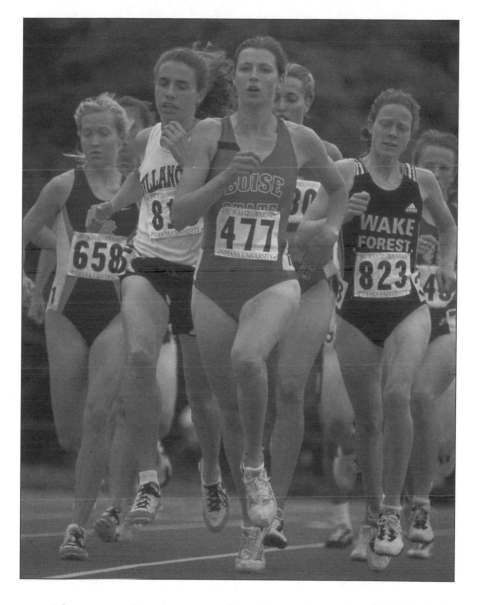

one of the main explanations as to why sodium citrate showed no ergogenic potential in the study done by Cox and Jenkins (1994) in which seven of the eight subjects experienced severe nausea. It was later suggested in the study that an abundance of water could help ease the gastrointestinal discomfort experienced during sodium citrate ingestion.

Tribulus 23

What Is It?

Tribulus terrestris, commonly known as the puncture vine, is an herbal preparation and has been used for centuries in Europe as a treatment for impotence and as sexual stimulant. For athletes, tribulus supposedly increases plasma testosterone, which therefore increases skeletal muscle mass. These effects, though, are unsubstantiated.

How Does It Work?

A study conducted by Dimitrov, Georgiev, and Vitanov (1987) could suggest an answer. They found that Tribestan (a tribulus-containing supplement) increased plasma testosterone levels in rams. This phenomenon theoretically occurs by stimulating the production of the luteinizing hormone, which is secreted from the brain (the pituitary gland to be specific). The luteinizing hormone consequently stimulates the testes to secrete the male sex hormone testosterone. The question that this study poses is, "Does this chain of events similarly occur in humans?" Let's examine some of the existing evidence to try to arrive at a conclusion.

The Evidence: Pro or Con?

The number of peer-reviewed studies on the effects of tribulus in weight-trained humans is sparse. There is only one known peer-reviewed study to date (Antonio, Uelmen et al. 2000). In that investigation, 15 healthy, resistance-trained men underwent an eight-week weight-training program coupled with daily supplementation of either a placebo or tribulus, 3.21 mg/kg body weight (or 1.5 mg/lb body weight). There were no changes in body weight, percentage body fat, total body water, or exercise performance. Though not significant, the placebo group had greater relative improvements in both muscular strength/endurance tests (see figure 23.1).

Guidelines for Use

At this point, there is no evidence that suggests tribulus affects plasma hormones (e.g., testosterone), lean body mass, or exercise performance. Future research should examine whether tribulus indeed has an effect on endocrine function. The claims made for this product—that it boosts both luteinzing hormone and testosterone levels—have simply never been substantiated.

Precautions

There were no reported side effects during the aforementioned eight-week study. Various combinations of doses and durations have yet to be studied.

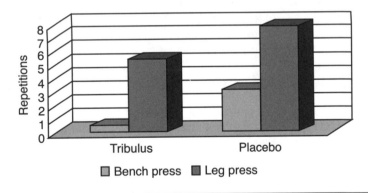

Figure 23.1 Average increase in total repetitions at 100% to 200% body weight. Adapted from Antonio, Uelmen et al. 2000

Vitamin C

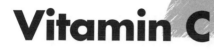

What Is It?

Vitamin C, also known as ascorbic acid, is a water-soluble vitamin found in many fruits and vegetables. It is one of the more important antioxidants present in the human body, but it cannot be endogenously synthesized by humans. Dietary deficiency of vitamin C leads to scurvy, a disease noted for a weakening in collagen-containing structures and ubiquitous capillary bleeding.

How Does It Work?

Vitamin C performs a myriad of functions in the body, many of which are vital to the athlete or active person. Its primary role is the synthesis of collagen, which is important for the strengthening of cartilage, tendons, and bones. Vitamin C also plays a critical role in the formation of neurotransmitters and hormones, both of which are released during exercise for the purpose of stimulating muscle growth and breaking down carbohydrates and fat for energy. In addition, vitamin C is involved in the synthesis of red blood cells, which are vital to delivering oxygen to the muscle. It is also a powerful antioxidant that prevents the buildup of free radicals in the body. Free radicals can lead to muscle and tendon damage as well as a host of other unwanted effects.

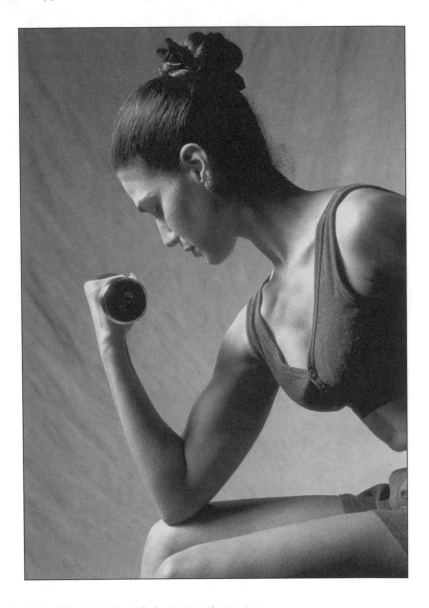

The Evidence: Pro or Con?

Supplementing vitamin C at doses between 500 and 3000 mg per day improves efficiency of submaximal workloads, increased peak work capacity, and increased muscular strength (Bramich et al. 1987; Howald et al. 1975). Recently, scientists at California State University in Fullerton examined the effects of vitamin C on the development of strength during eight weeks of weight training (Beam et al. 1998). Sixty-three subjects participated in this study and were split into two groups. Before testing, all members of both groups were tested for arm strength (biceps and triceps) and leg strength (quads and hamstrings). One group was given 1 g (1,000 mg) vitamin C per day while the other group was given a placebo. Both groups trained consistently during the eight-week testing period. The group taking vitamin C demonstrated significantly greater strength increases compared with the placebo group. It was concluded that vitamin C supplementation provides an advantage and results in a measurable improvement compared with taking nothing while weight training.

Guidelines for Use

More science needs to be done on vitamin C, but so far it would appear that 500 to 1,000 mg per day would benefit the strength-power athlete. Of course, it would behoove all athletes (and nonathletes as well) to consume a plethora of fruits and vegetables to get adequate vitamin C: broccoli, red and green peppers, berries, citrus fruits, and so on. However, it may be necessary to take supplemental vitamin C if the goal is to reach 500 to 1,000 mg per day.

Precautions

High doses of vitamin C may decrease the absorption of key minerals; it may cause diarrhea; or it may cause the development of kidney stones. Unfortunately, the scientific literature is not in complete agreement defining what a safe dose is. For instance, Johnston (1999) states that "the available data indicate that very high intakes of vitamin C (2-4 g/day) are well tolerated biologically in healthy mammalian systems." On the contrary, Levine et al. (1999) believe that ". . . the tolerable upper intake level is the highest daily level of nutrient intake that does not pose risk or adverse health effects to almost all individuals in the population. The amount is proposed to be less than 1 gram of vitamin C daily."

PART III

Supplement Combinations

The study of dietary supplements usually involves the detailed examination of single supplements in a double-blind, placebo-controlled fashion. Suffice to say that rarely do athletes or recreational fitness buffs take only singular supplements. For example, there are more than enough studies that show without a doubt that creatine has positive effects on performance and body composition. These studies, though, often use creatine in combination with carbohydrates, protein, or both. Additionally, you have other unique combinations to consider, such as zinc and magnesium, protein with added amino acids (e.g., glutamine), or caffeine plus ephedrine. In the real world, athletes stack supplements—that is, they use multiple supplements simultaneously—in what they term a "cycle." For instance, an athlete might consume a caffeine-ephedrine-aspirin stack during a two-week "on cycle" followed by a one-week "off cycle." Certainly, there are countless other combinations of cycling on and off a supplement. If you were to ask 100 athletes how they stack particular supplements, you may end up with 100 different answers.

The study of nutrient or supplement combinations, although criticized by scientists, may therefore actually be a better representation of what happens in the real world. Thus, in part II of this book, we discuss the effects of such combinations commonly used by athletes.

Colostrum, Creatine, Carnitine, and Coenzyme Q10

What Are They?

Colostrum (bovine) is a milk-like fluid secreted by mammals during the first few days after giving birth. It provides antibodies and growth factors that help support the development of the infant. Creatine is a methylglycocyamine that has consistently been shown to enhance anaerobic performance and increase lean body mass and muscle fiber area. Carnitine is a chemical that is involved in the oxidation of long-chain fatty acids, and coenzyme Q10—via aerobic metabolism—is involved in the generation of adenosine triphosphate (ATP), which is the "energy currency" of cells. (When ATP is split or hydrolyzed, energy is produced.)

How Do They Work?

Although the performance-enhancing effects of creatine are well-known, combining it with colostrum, carnitine, and coenzyme Q10 could theoretically provide further benefits. The question lies within the fact that any effect this combination has may be related to a synergism of two, three, or all of the ingredients. In other words, how do we know what combination was the one that produced the results? It would be difficult to parcel this information without extensive scientific investigation.

The Evidence: Pro or Con?

In a study from the University of Memphis, 49 resistance-trained subjects took part in a 12-week study that involved weight training plus dietary supplementation (Kerksick et al. 2001). There were four groups: (1) placebo (glucose); (2) colostrum; (3) Turbo ATP (1.5 g creatine, 1.5 g L-carnitine, 75 mg coenzyme Q10); and (4) colostrum plus the Turbo ATP. Supplements were isocaloric (same number of calories per serving), isonitrogenous (same levels of nitrogen from protein), and provided 60 g per day of casein/ whey (placebo group) or bovine colostrum. No significant differences were found for anaerobic sprint capacity or bench and leg press at one repetition maximum (1-RM); however, the change in bench press lifting volume was highest in the group that supplemented with the combination of colostrum plus Turbo ATP (see figure 25.1).

At the time of this writing, the aforementioned study was preliminary data and not yet published as a full-length scientific paper. Nonetheless, we can glean some interesting conclusions from this study. For instance, it is apparent that there is some sort of synergistic effect of colostrum with the Turbo ATP. Certainly, we know that creatine alone (which forms the basis of the Turbo product) can improve exercise performance. There is also preliminary evidence that colostrum may do the same. Perhaps they act via different mechanisms: For example, creatine might work via an increase in phosphocreatine (PCr) stores, and an increase in stored PCr would help in the regeneration of ATP. This chain of events could lead to an increase in available energy, and colostrum might therefore directly affect immune function, recovery, and so on. We could then reasonably conclude that colostrum acts synergistically as an ergogenic aid. At this

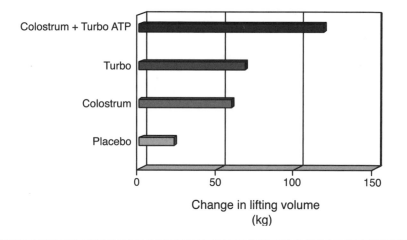

Change in lifting volume
(kg)

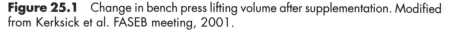

Figure 25.1 Change in bench press lifting volume after supplementation. Modified from Kerksick et al. FASEB meeting, 2001.

point, however, more research is needed to elucidate the exact workings of this combination.

Guidelines for Use

The available but limited data suggests that daily servings of colostrum (60 g), creatine (1.5 g), L-carnitine (1.5 g), and coenzyme Q10 (75 mg) may promote an ergogenic effect. It isn't known if there is a particular time one should take such a combination nor is it known if there are better combinations of these four nutrients.

Precautions

There are no known harmful effects regarding this specific combination of nutrients. Inasmuch as colostrum is the main part of this combination, it would be highly unlikely that this supplement could induce an ergolytic effect.

Creatine and β-Hydroxy-β-Methylbutyrate

What Are They?

Creatine is a nitrogenous organic compound that is synthesized to a small extent (2%) in the liver, pancreas, and kidneys from the amino acids arginine, methionine, and glycine (Pearson et al. 1999). Creatine can also be obtained through exogenous sources such as foods that are high in protein like fish and beef (Williams, Kreider, and Branch 1999). Approximately 95% of all the creatine stores in the body are found in skeletal muscle.

β-Hydroxy-β-methylbutyrate (HMB) is a breakdown product (metabolite) of the amino acid leucine (Nissen, Sharp et al. 1996). Leucine is found in all dietary protein and is an essential building block of protein in all tissues.

How Do They Work?

Creatine supplementation has been shown to increase total creatine and phosphocreatine (PCr) concentrations in skeletal muscle. This increase in creatine and PCr can improve the body's ability to generate energy via the increased capacity to resynthesize adenosine triphosphate (ATP). Some have also postulated that creatine supplementation increases cellular volume via an increase in intracellular water. This cellular swelling could augment protein synthesis.

HMB, on the other hand, has been shown to increase strength and lean body mass in exercising humans. HMB may have protein-sparing or anti-catabolic actions. Thus, the combination of these nutrients just may have a synergistic effect for the strength-power athlete.

The Evidence: Pro or Con?

In a recent study published in the journal *Nutrition* (Jowko et al. 2001), scientists examined the effects using a three-week supplementation program with four groups: One who supplemented with creatine only, 20 g daily for seven days followed by 10 g daily for 14 days; HMB only, 3 g daily; creatine and HMB, a combination of the two previously mentioned dosages; and a placebo. The subjects were 40 healthy males aged 19 to 23 who underwent a progressive resistance training program three times per week during the three-week treatment. They found that across all exercises, strength improved by 37.5, 39.1, and 51.9 kg in the HMB, creatine, and creatine plus HMB groups, respectively (see figure 26.1).

Guidelines for Use

According to this single investigation, combining 3 g HMB plus 10 to 20 g creatine daily for three weeks can improve strength more than taking either creatine or HMB as a single supplement. Although more research is needed to confirm this observation, there is plenty of evidence that both of these ingredients (as single supplements) are quite effective for augmenting performance in strength-power athletes.

Precautions

There are no harmful effects of this supplement combination according to aforementioned study. In fact, creatine and HMB have a plethora of data that shows them to be a safe and effective ergogenic aid.

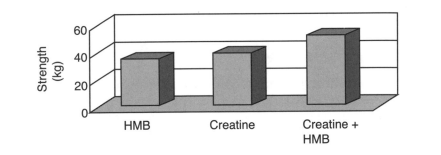

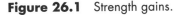

Figure 26.1 Strength gains.

Essential Amino Acids

27

What Are They?

Essential amino acids (EAA) are not made by the body and must be obtained through the diet. EAA include the following: isoleucine, leucine, valine, lysine, methionine, phenylalanine, threonine, and tryptophan. High levels of the essential amino acids can be found in any of a number of animal-based proteins (e.g., beef, pork, chicken, milk, egg, and so on).

How Do They Work?

Amino acids are the building blocks of protein in the body. They are essential for making structural proteins, enzymes, and certain hormones and neurotransmitters. Amino acids are also involved in metabolic pathways that affect exercise metabolism (Kreider 1999). In addition, it has also been suggested that additional protein (amino acids) in the diet may enhance muscle tissue growth and serve as a potential energy source during exercise (Kreider, Miriel, and Bertun 1993).

Recently, scientists have demonstrated that the consumption of EAA can augment muscle protein synthesis in healthy human subjects (Rasmussen et al. 2000; Tipton et al. 1999). For example, Dr. Tipton and colleagues at the University of Texas Medical Branch in Galveston, Texas, examined the effects of EAA in six healthy adults, three men and three women. The subjects participated in resistance exercise and followed it with the consumption of either 40 g EAA or a placebo. Investigators then examined the subjects' muscle protein synthesis and found that the acute ingestion of EAA was very effective at stimulating muscle protein anabolism. In a follow-up study using the same protocol (but with only 6 g EAA and 35 g sugar), Dr. Rasmussen and colleagues demonstrated a significantly greater anabolic drive—that is, the building of new muscle tissue—with the EAA supplement (when given after resistance exercise) versus the placebo supplement.

The Evidence: Pro or Con?

Dr. Maresh and colleagues (1991) performed a study on ATP-E, a supplement made of mostly EAA. The dose was 0.1 g ATP-E per kg of body weight (about 0.05/lb, or 10 g for a 200-lb person). The exact formula, using this dosage, is shown here.

L-glycine	0.12 mg/kg (0.05 mg/lb) body weight
L-arginine	0.47 mg/kg (0.21 mg/lb) body weight
D/L-methionine	2.33 mg/kg (1.06 mg/lb) body weight
L-aspartate	1.73 mg/kg (0.79 mg/lb) body weight
L-tryptophan	0.50 mg/kg (0.23 mg/lb) body weight
L-phenylalanine	0.41 mg/kg (0.19 mg/lb) body weight
L-histidine	0.39 mg/kg (0.18 mg/lb) body weight
L-proline	0.29 mg/kg (0.13 mg/lb) body weight
Choline chloride	1.96 mg/kg (0.89 mg/lb) body weight
Inositol	1.73 mg/kg (0.79 mg/lb) body weight
D-ribose	1.73 mg/kg (0.79 mg/lb) body weight
Magnesium phosphate	1.49 mg/kg (0.68 mg/lb) body weight

In their study, 23 active college male subjects performed six Wingate anaerobic power tests before ATP-E or placebo ingestion. At days 14 and 21, they performed the tests after supplementation. There were no significant differences between ATP-E and the placebo in peak power, mean power, rating of perceived exertion, and immediate postexercise heart rate. The results from this study show that 21 days of ATP-E supplementation had no effect on the strength-power.

In another study, Vukovich, Sharp et al. (1997) performed a study with untrained subjects for both aerobic and anaerobic training programs using the EAA called "branched-chain amino acids" (BCAA): valine, leucine, and isoleucine. Fourteen healthy, untrained college males participated. Body composition and performances were measured before supplementation, one week after supplementation, and at weeks two and six after starting supplementation with training. Subjects were given 2.9 g

BCAA supplement per day. Aerobic and anaerobic exercise was performed on the cycle ergometer Monday through Friday for the six weeks. The combination of BCAA with training demonstrated no significant changes in any of the performance and body composition measures. It was suggested that the small number of subjects and low dose of supplement may account for the lack of significance in this study.

More recently, Tipton et al. (2001) studied the effects of taking a combination of EAA (6 g) plus sucrose (35 g). The study examined whether taking it immediately before or immediately after had a differential impact on muscle protein metabolism. Interestingly, they discovered that if you consumed this mixture immediately before weight training, total net phenylalanine uptake across the leg, which is a measure of muscle protein accretion or gain, was more than double than if consumed immediately after weight training. An examination of figure 27.1 shows that this mixture taken before exercise is 158% better versus consumption after exercise.

Another study, conducted by Dr. Antonio and colleagues (Antonio, Sanders et al. 2000) examined the effects of six weeks of EAA supplementation on body composition and exercise performance in untrained women. Twenty-one subjects were given an average daily dose of 18.3 g EAA and participated in aerobic and resistance training three days per week. The resistance-training program consisted of split-routine, multiple-set training. The aerobic exercise consisted of 20 minutes at approximately 70% of the estimated maximum heart rate. The results of the study indicated no effect on body composition or muscular strength, but it did show significant differences in muscular endurance. Any changes

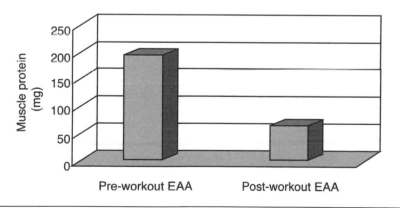

Figure 27.1 Muscle protein accretion when EAA are consumed before and after workouts.

that did occur in strength were found to be due to neural adaptation rather than muscle hypertrophy. Evidence from this study demonstrates that amino acid supplementation may not benefit a strength-training program, but it may assist endurance training.

Guidelines for Use

The available evidence from short-term studies using 6 to 40 g EAA given immediately before or after exercise suggests that it may potentiate the anabolic stimulus of exercise training. It is also possible that the consumption of EAA before exercising increases muscle protein synthesis more than if consumed postexercise. More evidence is needed to determine the long-term benefits of EAA supplementation.

Precautions

EEA are safe supplements. We hope that future research will parcel out the best or most ideal combination(s) of amino acids, carbohydrate, and even fat. However, high doses (>40 g) may result in gastrointestinal distress in certain athletes.

Phosphates and Creatine

28

What Are They?

Phosphate (or phosphorus) is a nonmetallic element, and following calcium, it is the most abundant mineral in the body. Accordingly, phosphates (as sodium or potassium phosphate) are extremely important in human metabolism. Approximately 80 to 90% of the phosphorus in the body combines to form calcium phosphate, which is used for the development of bones and teeth. Other phosphate salts, such as sodium phosphate, are involved in acid-base balance. The remainder of the body's phosphates are found in a variety of organic forms, including phospholipid, which help form cell membranes and DNA (part of the genetic material).

Additionally, phosphates are essential to the normal function of most of the B vitamins involved in the energy processes within the cell. Found in the muscle cell, phosphates are part of phosphocreatine and adenosine triphosphate (ATP, your cell's stored "energy currency"), which are high-energy compounds needed for muscle contraction. Glucose as well needs phosphates in order to be phosphorylated to proceed through glycolysis, which is a metabolic pathway that produces ATP. Finally, organic phosphates are part of a compound in red blood cells known as 2,3-DPG (2,3-diphosphoglycerate), which facilitates the release of oxygen to the muscle tissues (Bucci 1993).

Creatine (see pages 47-56), on the other hand, is a nitrogenous amine and occurs naturally in the body (mainly skeletal muscle) and in food such as beef, chicken, pork, and fish. Because creatine forms part of the phosphocreatine (PCr) molecule, it has been suggested that creatine supplementation can enhance intramuscular levels of this important compound. PCr is an important energy source for short-term, high-intensity exercise such as sprinting, jumping, or weightlifting.

How Does It Work?

The mechanism by which phosphate works is based on its ability to buffer lactic acid, improve the body's ability to deliver oxygen to contracting muscles, and enhance the cardiovascular system's ability to deliver more nutrients to the muscle, which is important for muscle growth. Creatine supplementation works by increasing creatine phosphate levels in the muscle, which allows for a greater anaerobic capacity. There is no doubt that creatine is probably the best and most effective supplement on the market, but it is the combination of phosphate and creatine that makes it a synergistic supplementation.

Here's how it works: When creatine is ingested, it enters the bloodstream as free creatine. To be trapped by the muscle cell, creatine must first be phosphorylated; that is, a phosphate is attached to it (the same goes for glucose to make glycogen). The amount of creatine that is phosphorylated is dependent on how much phosphate is available. The human body can only supply a limited amount, and unfortunately, it may not be enough. As a result, a lot of creatine may be lost during the loading phase. Furthermore, during intense exercise, muscle fatigue develops quickly because the ability to produce enough ATP for muscle contraction diminishes. The regeneration of ATP for repeated reps and sets in the gym then relies more on glycolysis and creatine phosphate. Therefore, it has been suggested that if phosphates can be provided to the muscles during intense exercise, it would delay the exhaustion of creatine phosphate stores.

The Evidence: Pro or Con?

Organic phosphate salt supplements, such as sodium and potassium phosphate, were reported to relieve fatigue in German soldiers during World War I. Other research in Germany during the 1930s suggested that phosphate salts actually improve physical performance (Bucci 1993).

A recent study (Wallace et al. 1997) investigated the effect of supplemental creatine alone versus creatine plus phosphate on muscle power. Male and female subjects were given either 5 g creatine four times per day or 5 g creatine plus 1 g phosphate four times per day for five days. The combination of creatine plus phosphate resulted in a significantly higher muscle power output, suggesting performance benefits more from a combination of phosphates and creatine than from creatine alone.

In agreement, Dr. Eckerson and colleagues (2001) at Creighton University examined the effects of creatine versus creatine plus phosphate on anaerobic working capacity (AWC). Male subjects were randomly put into one of three treatment groups: placebo (PL), 5 g creatine (Cr), or 5 g creatine plus 1 g phosphates (CrPh). Each subject was asked to dissolve their supplement in 16 oz water and ingest it four times per day for six consecutive days. The subjects performed a cycle ergometry test to determine AWC. The PL and Cr groups increased AWC by –3.0% and 16.0%, respectively. The CrPh group increased AWC by an incredible 49% (see figure 28.1).

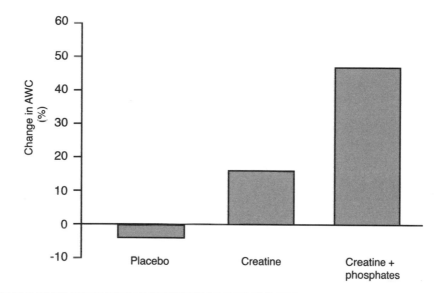

Figure 28.1 Effect of placebo, creatine, and creatine plus phosphates on performance.

Guidelines for Use

Taking phosphates with creatine may form a potent one-two punch. If you want to boost the effects of creatine, take a 1 g serving of phosphates (preferably a sodium-potassium mix) with every serving of creatine during the loading phase, which would be four times daily for 6 days. It is important that you do not take your phosphate with any dairy products.

Precautions

Dairy products such as milk, cheese, yogurt, and so on contain calcium, which could bind with the phosphates resulting in an upset stomach and poor absorption. According to Goss et al. (2001), there were no reported harmful effects of taking 4 g phosphate daily for two days in the form of potassium phosphate.

Whey Protein, Glutamine, and Branched-Chain Amino Acids

What Are They?

Whey is one of the proteins found in milk. Glutamine is a conditionally essential amino acid whereas the branched-chain amino acids (BCAA: valine, leucine, and isoleucine) are essential amino acids—that is, they must be consumed from foods or supplements. People do not usually require conditionally essential amino acids in their diet unless their bodies are subjected to greater than normal stress (e.g., illness, injury, prolonged exercise). When the body is subjected to such stress, its intake of a conditionally essential amino acid is higher.

How Do They Work?

An optimal diet is composed of adequate calories, protein, carbohydrates, and fat. Though a topic of intense debate, the use of protein supplements (versus simply consuming food) has often been proposed as a way to ensure the intake of high-quality protein. The use of amino acid supplements has also been touted as a way to improve body composition and athletic performance. So, the question is, Do whey, glutamine, and BCAA aid strength-power athletes better than or equal to a diet rich in protein? Let's briefly examine and explain each one's potential role.

First, whey is a complete protein—that is, it contains all of the essential amino acids—and it is rich in glutathione precursors (gamma-glutamylcysteine). There is data that shows that whey protein supplementation enhances longevity in mice (Bounous et al. 1989). Because of whey's role in modulating glutathione levels, it has been suggested that the regular consumption of whey may combat free radical damage and thus positively affect the level of oxidative damage induced by physical exercise.

Second, glutamine is the most abundant amino acid in plasma and skeletal muscle. Interestingly, it is used as the main fuel for various blood cells and the gastrointestinal tract. The exogenous supplementation of glutamine has been shown to have a protein-sparing effect as well as an immune-enhancing effect (Bounous and Gold 1991). The branched-chain amino acids (BCAA) also appear to prevent muscle degradation during prolonged exercise.

With regard to using a combination of any of these supplements, there is currently only one study that has examined the effects of combining whey protein, glutamine, and BCAA (Colker et al. 2000). We'll examine its findings closely in the following section.

The Evidence: Pro or Con?

One of the criticisms of the majority of studies published in the exercise science literature is the use of "untrained subjects" as the study group. First of all, untrained subjects are probably not going to be using supplements in the first place, and if they did, it would be in all likelihood a waste of time and money. Thus, it's always helpful when a study is published in which the study population comprises those who already exercise, preferably those who are already lifting weights.

In a study published in *Current Therapeutic Research* (Colker et al. 2000), scientists examined the effects of a combination of whey protein, glutamine, and BCAA on various physical parameters over a 10-week period in resistance-trained men (mean age 32). Sixteen men were divided into two groups and given daily supplements: One group received 40 g whey protein alone while the second group received 40 g whey protein plus 5 g glutamine and 3 g BCAA (1.5 g of leucine, 0.75 g valine, and 0.75 g isoleucine). Each subject followed a similar diet as instructed by a dietitian such that protein intake was kept at 1.6 g per kg of body weight per day (about 0.7 g/lb, or 140 g for a 200-lb person). Every subject participated in a supervised weight-training program geared toward promoting muscle hypertrophy (growth). Suffice it to say that the whey, glutamine, and BCAA group experienced much greater increases in muscular performance than the whey-only group. The physical test used was the maximum number of repetitions performed at 100% of body weight for bench press and 200% for leg press (see figure 29.1). The whey, glutamine, and BCAA group

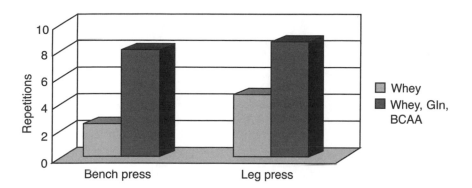

Figure 29.1 Increase in repetitions. Adapted from Colker et al. 2000.

improved more than double on average compared with the whey-only group.

Guidelines for Use

This single study suggests that daily supplementation of 40 g whey protein combined with 5 g glutamine and 3 g BCAA could induce an ergogenic effect. It isn't known if consuming such a stack, multiple times daily, would cause further alterations. We do know, however, that in addition to possible performance enhancement, the provision of extra protein and amino acids is a critical step toward increasing muscle mass and size. For certain athletes—like football players, bodybuilders, and weight lifters—the mere increase in muscle size should translate into improved muscular strength.

Precautions

There is no evidence that a combination of whey, glutamine, and BCAA as part of a dietary supplement has any deleterious effects. In fact, each of these supplements (taken alone) have been shown to have positive effects with little or no harmful effects.

Zinc-Magnesium Complex

What Is It?

Zinc (Zn) and magnesium (Mg) are two minerals that are needed for various metabolic processes. Zinc is a constituent of many enzymes involved in the major metabolic pathways; it is needed for normal digestion and the maintenance of hormonal levels. Magnesium, which can be found in over 300 enzymes, is prevalent in the body and is involved in energy production and various biosynthetic processes.

How Does It Work?

Children who are zinc-deficient are often growth-retarded and have reproductive system dysfunction. Zn supplementation can reverse these effects. (Also worth noting is that approximately 30% of adults may be Zn-deficient.) This deficiency is problematic in that plasma testosterone is regulated in part by Zn. Thus, a zinc deficiency may adversely affect this anabolic hormone, and as a consequence, it may have adverse effects on muscular mass and strength.

Magnesium, on the other hand, has been shown to decrease levels of the stress hormone cortisol (Golf et al. 1984). Excessive cortisol levels have an anti-catabolic effect on skeletal muscles (Crowley and Matt 1996). Therefore, supplementing with Mg may keep high levels of cortisol at bay, which would further allow the devopment of muscular mass and strength.

The Evidence: Pro or Con?

Part of the ergogenic effect of Zn or Mg is related to the fact that many of us do not consume sufficient levels of these important minerals. For example, serum zinc levels were "significantly below the normal range" in 23% of male and 43% of female athletes (Haralambie et al. 1981). Not only do most people not get enough of these minerals, but research has shown that runners and basketball players may actually *lose* zinc as a result of exercise (Lefavi et al. 1995). Therefore, whether in the form of supplements or food, athletes need to be aware of their Zn and Mg consumption to maintain healthy levels.

While zinc can be reasonably maintained through diet alone, magnesium may be more difficult to obtain from diet because the best sources are from unprocessed grains and nuts, foods not often found in the typical athlete's diet. In one study, 14 days of Mg aspartate supplementation (365 mg daily) was shown to decrease the amount of the stress hormone cortisol in the blood by 25% while subjects performed bike exercise (Golf et al. 1984). Thus, Mg theoretically has an anti-catabolic effect because high cortisol levels are known to promote muscle protein breakdown.

Perhaps the most telling study in favor of supplementing Zn and Mg is from the reputable *Journal of Exercise Physiology* (Brilla and Conte 2000). In a double-blind, placebo-controlled trial, 27 football players consumed daily either a placebo or a zinc-magnesium aspartate supplement (ZMA: 30 mg zinc monomethione aspartate, 450 mg magnesium aspartate, and 10.5 mg vitamin B6). Free testosterone and growth factor 1 (IGF-1) increased significantly in the ZMA-supplemented group but not in the placebo group (see figures 30.1 and 30.2). Strength, as measured with a Biodex dynamometer, improved more in the ZMA-supplemented group than in the placebo group (see table 30.1).

Table 30.1 Strength Changes After Zinc-Magnesium Supplementation

Group	Strength gain
ZMA	11-18%
Placebo	2-9%

Adapted from Brilla and Conte 2000.

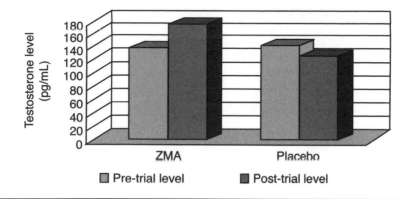

Figure 30.1 Changes in free testosterone. Adapted from Brilla and Conte 2000.

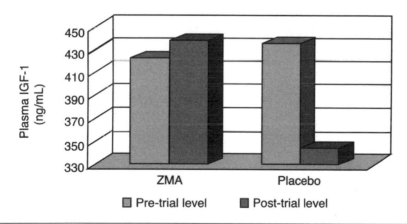

Figure 30.2 Changes in plasma IGF-1. Adapted from Brilla and Conte 2000.

Thus, the combination of Zn and Mg apparently has a positive influence on anabolic hormones and therefore improves exercise performance. Future studies need to confirm the ergogenic effects of this mineral combination. It is important to note that the Zn-Mg combination is found in the aspartate form in the Brilla study. Why is that so? Minerals bound to the amino acid aspartic acid are called "mineral aspartates." Aspartic acid functions as a transport mechanism for the mineral, which improves absorption.

Guidelines for Use

The recommended daily allowance (RDA) for Zn is 12 mg for women and 15 mg for men. The RDA for Mg is a dose of 280 mg for women and 350 mg for men. The Zn dose used in the Brilla study was 30 mg daily, so perhaps it would be wise not to exceed 30 mg daily for Zn. If you normally consume adequate Zn and Mg, it is not necessary to supplement.

Precautions

As a daily dietary supplement, do not exceed 15 to 30 mg zinc or 6 to 8 mg magnesium per kg body weight (6.8-13.6 mg zinc per lb; 2.7-3.6 mg magnesium per lb). Ingestion of 2 g or more Zn may cause vomiting and gastrointestinal irritation. Too much zinc can also adversely affect copper status and impair the immune system. If you have normal kidney function, there is no evidence that large oral intakes of Mg are harmful. As with most minerals, however, moderation is the key.

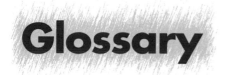

Glossary

ADP (Adenosine Diphosphate)—An essential chemical involved in the energy production of a cell. ADP is formed when ATP is broken down to supply energy for muscular contraction.

aerobic—Meaning "requiring oxygen." Aerobic metabolism happens during low-intensity, long-duration exercises.

"all natural"—Gym lingo to describe athletes who have not used anabolic steroids for a particular period of time. Natural athletic competitions are usually open to athletes who have not used steroids or other banned ergogenic aids for a period of no less than one year.

amino acids—A group of nitrogen-containing, carbon-based organic compounds that serve as the building blocks from which proteins (and muscle) are made.

anabolic—Referring to something that causes a buildup of tissue, or an anabolism. Anabolism generally refers to an increase in lean tissue, particularly muscle.

anabolic steroids—Synthetic versions of the male hormone testosterone. Anabolic steroids speed up protein synthesis, reduce catabolism, and increase strength and muscle mass in athletes who train with weights. They also may affect other parts of the body with serious side effects.

anaerobic—Anaerobic metabolism involves creating energy (ATP) without oxygen during explosive activities like weightlifting.

anti-catabolic—Referring to something that may prevent the breakdown of tissue (muscle).

antioxidants—May help control the damaging effects of free radicals.

anti-proteolysis—This is a specific type of anti-catabolism: Namely, the slowing or halting of protein (muscle) breakdown in the body.

ATP (Adenosine Triphosphate)—High-energy molecules stored in muscle and other cells in the body. When a muscle cell needs energy to contract, ATP is broken down to ADP to provide this energy. ATP can be thought of as the actual fuel that makes muscles move.

bioavailability—The ease with which something is absorbed from the digestive tract. The higher the bioavailability, the greater the total absorption and rate of absorption.

biological value (BV)—The BV score gives us an indication of how much of the protein eaten remains in the body (the rest is excreted via sweat, urine, and feces). Because the BV score is measured relative to a high-quality "test protein" (usually egg protein), the test protein is given a BV of 100. A BV score of 70% or greater is usually considered a high-quality protein.

buffer—A substance that minimizes changes in hydrogen-ion concentration (pH) such as sodium phosphate that athletes use to help reduce lactic-acid buildup during strenuous exercise.

carbohydrates—Organic compounds containing carbon, hydrogen, and oxygen. They're a very effective fuel source for the body. Types of carbohydrates include starches, sugars, and fibers, and each gram contains four calories. Carbohydrates are also classified into three groups: monosaccharides, disaccharides, and polysaccharides. Glucose (blood sugar) is a carbohydrate used by every cell in the body as fuel.

catabolism—Refers to the breakdown of tissue, particularly muscle.

chelating agent—An organic (hydrogen- and carbon-containing) compound that binds to charged metallic atoms (ions) to increase absorption.

cholesterol—A type of lipid that is a vital component in the production of many steroid hormones in the body; most widely known as a "bad fat," implicated as promoting heart disease and stroke.

coenzyme—An organic (hydrogen- and carbon-containing) compound that binds to a specific type of enzyme to activate it. A coenzyme is a type of cofactor. B vitamins commonly act as coenzymes.

cofactor—An inorganic substance that binds to a specific type of enzyme to activate it. Vitamins and minerals frequently serve as cofactors.

complete proteins—Proteins that contain all the essential amino acids.

creatine phosphate (CP)—CP donates the energy and the inorganic phosphate molecule that binds with ADP to form ATP. Supplementing with creatine monohydrate helps increase your muscle's CP reserves.

deficiency—A suboptimal level of one or more nutrients that are essential for good health. Most often seen with vitamins, a deficiency can be caused by poor nutrition or increased bodily demands, especially from intense training.

DEXA—"Dual-energy X-ray absorptiometry"; used to determine body composition. A good method for measuring body fat, lean body mass, and bone mineralization.

dextrose—Another name for glucose.

dipeptides—Protein fragments made up of only two amino acids.

disaccharide—A carbohydrate compound made up of two sugars.

double-blind study—An investigation in which neither the study participant nor the principal investigator or scientist is aware of the treatment(s) that the study participant is receiving.

effervescent—Producing and releasing gas bubbles. Effervescence provides a means of some drug or dietary supplement delivery systems and is intended to enhance absorption of the active ingredient(s).

efficacy—The maximum ability of a supplement to produce a desired result.

electrolytes—Substances that, in solution, are capable of conducting electricity. These charged particles are present throughout the body and are involved in many activities such as regulating the distribution of water inside and outside cells in the body.

endogenous—Originating from within the body; anything produced inside the body. For example, the hormone testosterone is endogenous.

engineered food—A kind of nutrition supplement that is designed to augment the diet or to replace a meal. It typically contains carbohydrate, fat, protein, vitamins, and minerals.

enzyme—A protein molecule that acts as a "helper" in thousands of chemical reactions in the body, such as digestion, hormone and energy production, muscle-cell repair, and so on.

ergogenic—Possessing the ability to enhance work output, particularly as it relates to athletic performance.

ergolytic—Possessing the ability to decrease work output. Sometimes what is intended to enhance physical performance inadvertently hinders performance.

exogenous—Refers to the substances that are introduced into the body. For example, an exogenous dose of anabolic steroids would refer to steroids given orally or via injection. This is in contrast with endogenous steroids, which are naturally produced by the endocrine system.

fat—One of the macronutrients. Fat contains nine calories per gram; it has the most calories of all macronutrients. Dietary fats may also be referred to as lipids or triglycerides. Fats serve a variety of functions in the body. For example, they act as structural components for all cell membranes, as well as supply necessary chemical substrates for hormone production. There are two types of fat—saturated ("bad") and unsaturated ("good").

fat-free mass (FFM)—All portions of body tissues not containing fat, such as bones, muscles, skin, and organs, in addition to body water, hair, blood, and lymph.

free radicals—A highly reactive atom or compound having an unpaired electron. Free radicals are produced during metabolism (energy creation) and are believed to cause cellular damage. Free radicals may play a role in aging and disease.

fructose—The main type of sugar found in fruit. Sweeter than table sugar, it is often used as a sugar substitute for diabetics.

full-spectrum amino acids—Supplements that contain a combination of all the essential amino acids.

glucagon—A hormone that is responsible for helping maintain proper blood sugar levels by breaking down glycogen to glucose.

glucose—The simplest sugar molecule. It's the main sugar found in blood and is used as a basic fuel for the body. Too much glucose causes your body to release a rapid and large amount of insulin to counteract the large influx of sugar.

glucose disposal agent—A nutrient or complex of nutrients that has the ability to increase insulin sensitivity, thus allowing circulating blood glucose to be readily deposited into target tissues.

glycemic index (GI)—A measure of the extent to which a food raises the blood sugar (glucose) level as compared with white bread or glucose, which has a GI of 100.

glycogen—The principal storage form of carbohydrate energy (glucose), which is stored in muscles and in the liver.

growth hormone (GH)—An anabolic hormone naturally released by the pituitary gland. GH promotes muscle growth and the breakdown of body fat for energy.

HDL—Stands for "high-density lipoprotein." It's one of the subcategories of cholesterol, typically thought of as the "good" cholesterol.

hormones—Molecules, either protein or steroids, that regulate various biological processes in the body.

hypertrophy—Meaning to increase in size.

hypoglycemia—A low blood sugar / glucose level, which results in anxiety, fatigue, perspiration, delirium, and in severe cases, coma. Mostly occurring in diabetics. When it occurs in athletes, it can be overcome with the ingestion of carbohydrates.

insulin—An anabolic hormone secreted by the pancreas that aids the body in maintaining proper blood sugar levels and promoting glycogen storage. Insulin secretion speeds the movement of nutrients through the bloodstream and into muscle for growth.

insulin amplifier—A nutrient or complex of nutrients that has the ability to increase the secretion of insulin.

lactic acid—A molecule produced from glucose during anaerobic metabolism. When oxygen becomes available, lactic acid can be completely broken down to carbon dioxide and water. Lactic-acid buildup is a primary cause of muscle fatigue. Supplements that limit lactic-acid buildup may enhance athletic performance.

LDL—Stands for "low-density lipoprotein" and is a subcategory of cholesterol, typically thought of as the "bad" cholesterol. LDL is the type of cholesterol that circulates throughout the bloodstream and may cause heart disease.

lean body mass (LBM)—Another term that describes fat-free mass.

lipid—Another name for dietary fats or triglycerides.

lipogenic—Literally translated as "fat producing"; that is, it means to make body fat.

lipolysis—The chemical breakdown of body fat by enzymes that results in stored body fat being used as fuel by the body.

luteinizing hormone (LH)—A powerful hormone that (in men) stimulates the testes to make testosterone and (in women) induces ovulation.

meal-replacement powders (MRPs)—A category of supplements that contain protein, carbohydrates, vitamins, minerals, and other key nutrients. They are used to replace regular food for purposes of weight loss, weight gain, or increasing dietary nutrient intake.

metabolic rate—The rate you convert energy stores into working energy in the body. In other words, it's how fast your whole system runs. The metabolic rate is controlled by a number of factors, such as caloric intake, exercise, the use of stimulant or depressant chemicals, and muscle mass (the greater your muscle mass, the greater your metabolic rate).

metabolite—Any product of metabolism, such as an intermediate or waste product. For example, the popular supplement HMB is a metabolite (a breakdown product) of the amino acid leucine.

nitrogen—An element that distinguishes proteins from other substances and allows them to form various structural units in our bodies, including enzymes and muscle proteins.

nitrogen balance—When a person's daily intake of nitrogen from proteins equals the daily excretion of nitrogen.

nutraceuticals—Substances in a food that may provide medical or health benefits beyond basic nutrition, including disease prevention.

nutrients—Components of food that help nourish the body; that is, they provide energy or serve as "building materials." These nutrients include carbohydrates, fats, proteins, vitamins, minerals, water, and so on.

patent—A numeric distinction granted to an invention by the U.S. Patent Office. A patent gives exclusive rights, or a monopoly, to the inventor for production, use, sale, and profit. In regard to dietary supplements, a patent signifies only that a product is unique, not that it is effective.

peptide—A compound made up of two or more amino acids. Protein molecules are broken down into peptides in the intestines and absorbed in that form.

pharmaceutical grade—Implying purity. This term has no legal or trade definition but is frequently used on sports supplement labels.

phytochemical—Substances found in fruits and vegetables that exhibit a potential for reducing risk of cancer.

placebo—A harmless, inactive substance that may be given in the place of an effective drug or substance, especially to control groups in clinical studies.

polysaccharides—Carbohydrates containing a large number of sugar groups. Starch, glycogen, dextrin, and cellulose are examples.

power—The amount of work an individual can perform in a given period of time.

precursors—Compounds from which another compound is formed in the body. For example, choline is a precursor to acetylcholine, a neurotransmitter involved in muscle contraction.

proteins—Highly complex nitrogen-containing compounds found in all animal and vegetable tissues. They are made up of amino acids and are essential for growth and repair in the body. A gram of protein contains four calories. Those from animal sources are high in biological value because they contain essential amino acids. Those from vegetable sources contain some, but not all, of the essential amino acids. Proteins are the building blocks of muscle, enzymes, and some hormones.

pure—Referring to a supplement that contains nothing but the ingredients stated on the label. This term has no legal definition.

saturated fats—"Bad" fats. They are called "saturated" because they contain no open spots on their "carbon skeletons." Saturated fats include myristic acid, palmitic acid, stearic acid, arachidic acid, and lignoceric acid, which have been shown to raise cholesterol levels in the body. Sources of these fats include animal foods and hydrogenated vegetable oils such as margarine. These fats serve no biological function in the body, other than to supply calories.

stacking—Consumption of two or more supplements during the same time frame in an attempt to maximize results. This term originated with anabolic steroid regimens.

strength—The amount of weight one can lift with one repetition.

sublingual—Meaning "beneath the tongue." Several supplements available to athletes are made to be taken in this manner.

sucrose—Most commonly known as table sugar. Industrially, sucrose is derived from sugar cane or sugar beets. When you eat it, the body breaks sucrose into fructose and glucose; consequently, it has some of the properties of fructose and glucose. Eating it elicits a rapid insulin response but not as high as one caused by glucose.

synergistic—Having the property of enhancing or multiplying the effectiveness of another substance. For example, carbohydrates consumed with creatine monohydrate may have a synergistic relationship.

testosterone—The anabolic hormone that makes muscles grow, produced primarily by the testes in men. It biologically separates the men from the boys.

thermogenic—To speed up the metabolism, raise core body temperature, and accelerate calorie expenditure.

triglyceride—The scientific name for a common dietary fat. The backbone of this molecule is a glycerol molecule that is connected to three fatty acid molecules. Triglycerides are also called fats or lipids.

tripeptide—Protein fragments that are the length of three amino acids.

unsaturated fats—"Good" fats. They are called unsaturated because they have one or more open carbon spots. Unsaturated fats can be divided into two categories: polyunsaturated and monounsaturated. Unsaturated fats have been shown to help reduce cholesterol and triglyceride levels in the blood. This category of fats includes the essential fatty acids linoleic acid and alpha-linolenic acid.

vitamins—Organic compounds that are vital to life, indispensable to bodily function, and needed in minute amounts. They are noncaloric essential nutrients. Many of them function as coenzymes, supporting a multitude of biological functions.

$\dot{V}O_2$ **max**—The maximum volume of oxygen an individual can consume per minute of work. It is often used to evaluate an athlete's cardiovascular efficiency and thus performance capacity.

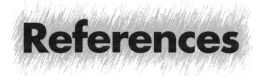

References

Agnusdei, D., et al. 1997a. A double-blind, placebo-controlled trial of ipriflavone for prevention of postmenopausal spinal bone loss. *Calcified Tissue International* 61:142-47.

Agnusdei, D., et al. 1997b. Efficacy of ipriflavone in established osteoporosis and long-term safety. *Calcified Tissue International* 61, suppl. 1:S23-27.

Almada, A., R. Kreider, M. Ferreira, and M. Wilson. 1997. Effects of calcium B-HMB supplementation with or without creatine during training on strength and sprint capacity. *Federation of American Societies for Experimental Biology* 11:A376.

Anselme, F., K. Collomp, B. Mercier et al. 1992. Caffeine increases maximal anaerobic power and blood lactate concentration. *European Journal of Applied Physiology* 65:188-91.

Antonio, J., and C. Street. 1999. Glutamine: A potentially useful supplement for athletes. *Canadian Journal of Applied Physiology* 24:1-14.

Antonio, J., D. Falk, and D. Van Gammeren. 2001. Ribose supplementation improves muscular strength and endurance in male bodybuilders. *Federation of American Societies for Experimental Biology Journal* 15(5):A752 (March).

Antonio, J., J. Uelmen, R. Rodriguez, and C. Earnest. 2000. The effects of Tribulus Terrestris on body composition and exercise performance in resistance-trained males. *International Journal of Sport Nutrition and Exercise Metabolism* 10:208-15.

Antonio, J., M. Sanders, L. Ehler, J. Uelmen, J. Raether, and J. Stout. 2000. Effects of exercise training and amino acid supplementation on body composition and physical performance in untrained women. *Nutrition* 16:1-4.

Antonio, J., M.S. Sanders, and D. Van Gammeren. 2001. The effects of bovine colostrum supplementation on body composition and exercise performance in active men and women. *Nutrition* 17(3):243-47.

Antonio, J., T. Incledon, and D. Van Gammeren. 2000. The effects of 5-methyl-7-methoxyisoflavone on body composition and performance in college-aged men. *Journal of Performance Enhancement* (online).

Ball, D., and R.J. Maughan. 1997. The effect of sodium citrate ingestion on the metabolic response to intense exercise following diet manipulation in man. *Experimental Physiology* 82:1041-56.

Balsom, P.D., B. Ekblom, K. Soderlund, B. Sjodin, and E. Hultman. 1993. Creatine supplementation and dynamic intensity intermittent exercise. *Scandinavian Journal of Medicine in Science and Sport* 3:143-49.

Beam, W.C., et al. 1998. The effect of chronic ascorbic acid supplementation on strength following isotonic strength training. *Medicine and Science in Sports and Exercise* 30:S219.

Becque, M.D., J.D. Lochmann, and D.R. Melrose. 2000. Effects of oral creatine supplementation on muscle strength and body composition. *Medicine and Science in Sports and Exercise* 32:654-58.

Bidzinska, B., F. Petraglia, S. Angioni et al. 1993. Effect of different chronic intermittent stressors and acetyl-l-carnitine on hypothalamic beta-endorphin and GnRH and on plasma testosterone levels in male rats. *Neuroendocrinology* 57:985-90.

Bigard, A.X., P. Lavier, L. Ullmann et al. 1996. Branched-chain amino acid supplementation during repeated prolonged skiing exercises at altitude. *International Journal of Sport Nutrition* 6:295-306.

Birch, R., D. Noble, and P.L. Greenhaff. 1994. The influence of dietary creatine supplementation on performance during repeated bouts of maximal isokinetic cycling in man. *European Journal of Applied Physiology* 69 (3):268-76.

Blomqvist, B.I., F. Hammarqvist, A. von der Decken, and J. Wernerman. 1995. Glutamine and alpha-ketoglutarate prevent the decrease in muscle free glutamine concentration and influence protein synthesis after total hip replacement. *Metabolism* 44:1215-22.

Bogodanis, G.C., M.E. Nevill, H.K. Lakomy, B. H. Boobis. 1998. Power output and muscle metabolism during and following recovery from 10 and 20 s of maximal sprint exericse in humans. *Acta Physiol Scand* 163(3):261-72.

Bounous, G., and P. Gold. 1991. The biological activity of undenatured dietary whey proteins: Role of glutathione. *Clinical and Investigative Medicine* 14(4):296-309.

Bounous, G., F. Gervais, V. Amer et al. 1989. The influence of dietary whey protein on tissue glutathione and the diseases of aging. *Clinical Investigative Medicine* 12:343-49.

Bowtell, J.L., et al. 1999. Effect of oral glutamine on whole body carbohydrate storage during recovery from exhaustive exercise. *Journal of Applied Physiology* 86:1770-77.

Bramich, K., et al. 1987. The effects of two levels of ascorbic acid on muscular endurance, muscular strength and on $\dot{V}O_2$ max. *International Clinical Nutrition Review* 7:5.

Brilla, L.R., and V. Conte. 2000. Effects of a novel zinc-magnesium formulation on hormones and strength. *Journal of Exercise Physiology* (online) 3 (4):26-36.

Broeder, C.E., J. Quindry, K. Brittingham et al. 2000. The Andro Project: Physiological and hormonal influences of androstenedione supplementation in men 35 to 65 years old participating in a high-intensity resistance training program. *Archives of Internal Medicine* 160:3093-3104.

Bucci, L. 1993. *Nutrients as ergogenic aids for sports and exercise.* Boca Raton, Fla.: CRC Press.

Buckley, J., et al. 1998. Effect of oral bovine colostrum supplement (Intact) on running performance. Proceedings of the Australian Conference of Science and Medicine in Sport, October. 79.

Buckley, J., et al. 2001. Effect of bovine colostrum supplementation on the composition of resistance trained and non-trained limbs. *Medicine and Science in Sports and Exercise* 33(5):S340 (abstract for 2001 ACSM national meeting).

Buckspan, R., B. Hoxworth, E. Cersosimo, J. Devlin, E. Horton, and N. Abumrad. 1986. A-Ketoisocarpoate is superior to leucine in sparing glucose utilization in man. *American Journal of Physiology* 251:E648-53.

Burke, E.R. 1999. *D-Ribose: What you need to know.* Garden City Park, NY: Avery Publishing Group.

Candeloro, N., I. Bertini, G. Melchiorri, and A. De Lorenzo. 1995. Effects of prolonged administration of branched-chain amino acids on body composition and physical fitness. *Minerva Endocrinol* 20:217-23.

Candow, D.G., P.D. Chilibeck, D.G. Burke, and K.S. Davison. 2000. Effect of glutamine supplementation combined with resistance training. *Canadian Journal of Applied Physiology* 25 (5):363.

Casey, A.D., S. Constantin-Teodosiu, S. Howell, E. Hultman, and P.L. Greenhaff. 1996. Creatine ingestion favorably affects performance and muscle metabolism during maximal exercise in humans. Part 1. *American Journal of Physiology* 271 (1):E31-37.

Castell, L.M., and E.A. Newsholme. 1998. Glutamine and the effects of exhaustive exercise upon the immune response. *Canadian Journal of Physiology and Pharmacology* 76 (5):524-32.

Castell, L.M., J. R. Poortmans, and E.A. Newsholme. 1996. Does glutamine have a role in reducing infections in athletes? *European Journal of Applied Physiology* 73:488-90.

Cerosimo, E., B.M. Miller, W.W. Lacy, and N. Abrumrad. 1983. A-Ketoisocaproate, not leucine, is responsible for nitrogen sparing during progressive fasting in normal male volunteers. *Surgical Forum* 34:96-98.

Chetlin, R.D., R.A. Yeater, I.H. Ullrich et al. 2000. The effect of ornithine alpha-ketoglutarate (OKG) on healthy, weight-trained men. *Journal of Exercise Physiology* (online) 3, no. 4 (October).

Chua, B., D.L. Siehl, and H.E. Morgan. 1979. Effect of leucine and metabolites of branched chain amino acids on protein turnover in heart. *Journal of Biological Chemistry* 254:8358-62.

Clancy, S., et al. 1994. Effects of chromium picolinate supplementation on body composition, strength and urinary chromium loss in football players. *International Journal of Sports Nutrition* 4:142-53.

Colker, C.M., et al. 2000. Effects of supplemental protein on body composition and muscular strength in healthy athletic adult males. *Current Therapeutic Research* 61:19-28.

Colker, C.M., J. Antonio, and D. Kalman. 2001. The metabolism of orally ingested 19-nor-4-androstene-3,17-dione and 19-nor-4-androstene-3,17-diol in healthy, resistance-trained men. *Journal of Strength and Conditioning Research* 15:144-47.

Collomp, K., S. Ahmaidi, M. Audran et al. 1991. Effects of caffeine ingestion on performance and anaerobic metabolism during the Wingate test. *International Journal of Sports Medicine* 12:439-43.

Collomp, K., S. Ahmaidi, J.C. Chatard et al. 1992. Benefits of caffeine ingestion on sprint performance in trained and untrained swimmers. *European Journal of Applied Physiology* 64:377-80.

Coombes, J., and L. McNaughton. 1993. Effects of bicarbonate ingestion on leg strength and power during isokinetic knee flexion and extension. *Journal of Strength and Conditioning Research* 7:241-49.

Cox, G., and D.G. Jenkins. 1994. The physiological and ventilatory responses to repeated 60s sprints following sodium citrate ingestion. *Journal of Sports Sciences* 12:469-75.

Crowley, M.A., and K.S. Matt. 1996. Hormonal regulation of skeletal muscle hypertrophy in rats: The testosterone to cortisol ratio. *European Journal of Applied Physiology* 73 (1-2):66-72.

Dalton, R.A., J.W. Rankin, D. Sebolt, and F. Gwazdauskas. 1999. Acute carbohydrate consumption does not influence resistance exercise performance during energy restriction. *International Journal of Sport Nutrition* 9:319-32.

Dangott, B., E. Schultz, and P. Mozdziak. 2000. Dietary creatine monohydrate supplementation increases satellite cell mitotic activity during compensatory hypertrophy. *International Journal of Sports Medicine* 21 (1):13-16.

De Bandt, J.P., C. Coudray-Lucas, N. Lioret et al. 1998. A randomized trial of the influence of the mode of enteral ornithine alpha-ketoglutarate administration in burn patients. *Journal of Nutrition* 128:563-69.

Demant, T.W., and E. Rhodes. 1999. Effects of creatine supplementation on exercise performance. *Sports Medicine* 28 (1):49-60.

Dimitrov, M., P. Georgiev, and S. Vitanov. 1987. Use of tribestan on rams with sexual disorders. *Veterinarnomeditsinski Nauki* 24 (5):102-10.

Earnest, C.P., M.A. Olson, C.E. Broeder, K. Bruel, and S.G. Beckman. 2000. Oral 4-androstene-3,17-dione and 4-androstene-3,17-diol supplementation in young males. *European Journal of Applied Physiology* 81:229-32.

Earnest, C.P., P.G. Snell, R. Rodriguez, A.L. Almada, and T.L. Mitchell. 1995. The effect of creatine monohydrate ingestion on anaerobic power indices, muscular strength and body composition. *Acta Physiol Scandinavica* 153 (2):207-9.

Eckerson, J., et al. 2001. The effect of creatine phosphate supplementation on anaerobic working capacity following 2 and 6 d of loading in men. Presented at the National Strength and Conditioning Association's national convention in Spokane, WA.

Edwards, M., E. Rhodes, D. McKenzie, and A. Belcastro. 2000. The effect of creatine supplementation on anaeorbic performance in moderately active men. *Journal of Strength and Conditioning Research* 14 (1):75-79.

Evans, G. 1996. *Chromium picolinate: Everything you need to know.* New York: Avery Publishing Group.

Ferrando, A.A., and N.R. Green. 1993. The effect of boron supplementation on lean body mass, plasma testosterone levels, and strength in male bodybuilders. *International Journal of Sport Nutrition* 3:140-49.

Feuer, L., et al. 1979. Metabolic 5-methyl-isoflavone-derivatives, process for preparation thereof and compositions containing the same. United States Patent 4,163,746. August 7, 1979.

Flakoll, P.J., M.H. Vandehaar, G. Kuhlman, S. Nissen. 1991. Influence of alpha-ketoisocaproate on lamb growth, feed conversion, and body composition. *Journal of Animal Science* 69 (4):1461-7.

Frayn, K.N., K. Khan, S.W. Coppack et al. 1991. Amino acid metabolism in human subcutaneous adipose tissue in vivo. *Clinical Science* 80:471-74.

Gaitanos, G., M. Nevill, S. Brooks, and C. Williams. 1991. Repeated bouts of sprint running after induced alkalosis. *Journal of Sports Sciences* 9:355-70.

Gaitanos, G.C., C. Williams, L.H. Boobis, and S. Brooks. 1993. Human muscle metabolism during intermittent maximal exercise. *Journal of Applied Physiology* 75 (2):712-19.

Gallagher, P.M., J.A. Carrithers, M.P. Godard, K.E. Schulze, and S.W. Trappe. 2000a. B-hydroxy-B-methylbutyrate ingestion, part I: Effects on strength and fat free mass. *Medicine and Science in Sports and Exercise* 32:2109-15.

Gallagher, P.M., J.A. Carrithers, M.P. Godard, K.E. Schulze, and S.W. Trappe. 2000b. B-hydroxy-B-methylbutyrate ingestin, part II: Effects on hematology, hepatic and renal function. *Medicine and Science in Sports and Exercise* 32:2116-19.

Gallagher, P.M., D.L. Williamson, M.P. Godard, J. Witter, S.W. Trappe. 2000c. Effects of ribose supplementation on adenine nucleotide concentration in skeletal muscle following high-intensity exercise. Paper presented at the Midwest Regional Chapter of the ACSM, October.

Gennari, C., et al. 1998. Effect of ipriflavone—a synthetic derivative of natural isoflavones—on bone mass loss in the early years after menopause. *Menopause* 5(1):9-15.

Gilliam, J., C. Hohzorn, D. Martin, and M. Trimble. 2000. Effect of oral creatine supplementation on isokinetic torque production. *Medicine and Science in Sports and Exercise* 32 (5):993-96.

Golf, S.W., et al. 1984. Plasma aldosterone, cortisol, and electrolyte concentrations in physical exercise after magnesium supplementation. *Journal of Clinical Chemistry and Clinical Biochemistry* 22:717-21.

Goss, F., et al. 2001. Effect of potassium phosphate supplementation on perceptual and physiological responses to maximal graded exercise. *International Journal of Sport Nutrition and Exercise Metabolism* 11:53-62.

Green, A.L., et al. 1996. Carbohydrate feeding augments creatine retention during creatine feeding in humans. *American Journal of Physiology* 271:E821-26.

Greenhaff, P.L., et al. 1993. The influence of oral creatine supplementation on muscle physphocreatine resynthesis following intense contraction in man. Abstract. *Journal of Physiology* 467:75P.

Greenhaff, P.L., K. Bodin, K. Soderlund, and E. Hultman. 1994. Effect of oral creatine supplementation on skeletal muscle phosphocreatine resynthesis. Part 1. *American Journal of Physiology* 266 (5):E725-30.

Greer, F., C. McLean, and T.E. Graham. 1998. Caffeine, performance, and metabolism during repeated Wingate exercise tests. *Journal of Applied Physiology* 85:1502-8.

Hannan, M.T., K.L. Tucker, B. Dawson-Hughes et al. 2000. Effect of dietary protein on bone loss in elderly men and women: The Framingham Osteoporosis Study. *Journal of Bone Mineral Research* 15:2504-12.

Haralambie, G., et al. 1981. Serum zinc in athletes in training. *International Journal of Sports Medicine* 2 (3):135-8.

Harris, R.C., K. Soderlund, and E. Hultman. 1992. Elevation of creatine in resting and exercised muscle of normal subjects by creatine supplementation. *Clinical Science* 83 (3):367-74.

Hausswirth, C., A.X. Bigard, R. Lepers, M. Berthelot, and C.Y. Guezennec. 1995. Sodium citrate ingestion and muscle performance in acute hypobaric hypoxia. *European Journal of Applied Physiology* 71:362-68.

Horswill, C., D. Costill, W. Fink, M. Flynn, J. Kirwan, J. Mitchell, and J. Houmard. 1988. Influence of sodium bicarbonate on sprint performance: Relationship to dosage. *Medicine and Science in Sports and Exercise* 20:566-69.

Howald, H., et al. 1975. Ascorbic acid and athletic performance. *Annals of the New York Academy of Sciences* 258:458-64

Hultman, E., and P.L. Greenhaff. 1991. Skeletal muscle energy metabolism and fatigue during intense exercise in man. *Science Progress* 75 (298):361-70.

Ibanez, J., T. Pullinen, E. Gorostiaga, A. Postigo, and A. Mero. 1995. Blood lactate and ammonia in short-term anaerobic work following induced alkalosis. *The Journal of Sports Medicine and Physical Fitness* 35:187-93.

Johnston, C.S. 1999. Biomarkers for establishing a tolerable upper intake level for vitamin C. *Nutrition Review* 57:71-77.

Jowko, W., et al. 2001. Creatine and beta-hydroxy-beta-methylbutyrate (HMB) additively increase lean body mass and muscle strength during a weight-training program. *Nutrition* 17:558-66.

Kalmar, J.M., and E. Cafarelli. 1999. Effects of caffeine on neuromuscular function. *Journal of Applied Physiology* 87:801-8.

Kelly, V.G., and D.G. Jenkins. 1998. Effect of oral creatine supplementation on near-maximal strength and repeated sets of high-intensity bench press exercise. *Journal of Strength and Conditioning Research* 12:109-115.

Kerksick, C., et al. 2001. Effects of bovine colostrum supplementation on training adaptations II: Performance. *Federation of American Societies for Experimental Biology Journal* 15(5):LB317.

King, D.S., R.L. Sharp, M.D. Vukovich et al. 1999. Effect of oral androstenedione on serum testosterone and adaptations to resistance training in young men: A randomized controlled trial. *Journal of the American Medical Association* 281 (21):2020-28.

Kirksey, K.B., M.H. Stone, B.J. Warren et al. 1999. The effects of 6 weeks of creatine monohydrate supplementation on performance measures and body composition in collegiate track and field athletes. *Journal of Strength and Conditioning Research* 13:148-156.

Kishikawa, Y., et al. 1996. Purification and characterization of cell growth factor in bovine colostrum. *Journal of Veterinarian Medicine Science* 58:47-53.

Kowalchuk, J.M., S.A. Maltais, K. Yamaji, and R.L. Hughson. 1989. The effect of citrate loading on exercise performance, acid-base balance and metabolism. *European Journal of Applied Physiology* 58:858-64.

Kraemer, W.J., et al. 1996. Strength and power training: Physiological mechanisms of adaptation. In *Exercise and sports science reviews*, edited by J.O. Holloszy, 363-97. Vol. 25. Baltimore: Williams and Wilkins.

Kraemer, W.J., and J. Volek. 1999. Creatine supplementation. Its role in human performance. *Clinical Sports Medicine* 18(3):651-66.

Kreider, R., V. Miriel, and E. Bertun. 1993. Amino acid supplementation and exercise performance. *Sports Medicine* 16:190-209.

Kreider, R.B. 1999. Effects of protein and amino acid supplementation on athletic performance. *Sportscience*. [Online]. Available: sportsci.org/jour/9901/rbk.html.

Kreider, R.B., M. Ferreira, M.Wilson, and A.L. Almada. 1997. Effects of calcium HMB supplementation with or without creatine during training on body composition alterations. *Federation of American Societies for Experimental Biology Journal* 11:A374.

Kreider, R.B., M. Ferreira, M. Wilson, and A.L. Almada. 1999. Effects of calcium beta-hydroxy-beta-methylbutyrate (HMB) supplementation during resistance training on markers of catabolism, body composition and strength. *International Journal of Sports Medicine* 20 (8):503-9.

Kreider, R.B., M. Ferreira, M. Wilson et al. 1998. Effects of creatine supplementation on body composition, strength, and sprint performance. *Medicine and Science in Sport and Exercise* 30 (1):73-82.

Kuhne, S., et al. 2000. Growth performance, metabolic and endocrine traits, and absorptive capacity in neonatal calves fed either colostrums or milk replacer at two levels. *Journal of Animal Science* 78:609-20.

Kuiper, G.G., et al. 1998. Interaction of estrogenic chemicals and phytoestrogens with estrogen receptor beta. *Endocrinology* 139:4252-63.

Kuipers, H., et al. 2001. Colostrum has no effect on growth factors and on a doping test. *Medicine and Science in Sports and Exercise* 33(5): S332.

Lacey, J.M., and D.W. Wilmore. 1990. Is glutamine a conditionally essential amino acid? *Nutrition Reviews* 48:297-309.

Lefavi, R.G., et al. 1992. Efficacy of chromium supplementation in athletes: Emphasis on anabolism. *International Journal of Sport Nutrition* 2(2):111-22.

Lefavi, R.G., et al. 1995. Reduced serum mineral levels in basketball players after season. *Medicine and Science in Sports and Exercise* 27(5): abstract.

Lemon, P.W. 1998. Effects of exercise on dietary protein requirements. *International Journal of Sport Nutrition* 8(4):426-47.

Lemon, P.W. 2000. Beyond the zone: Protein needs of active individuals. *Journal of the American College of Nutrition* 19 (5):513S-521S.

Lemon P.W., et al. 1997. Moderate physical activity can increase dietary protein needs. *Canadian Journal of Applied Physiology* 22 (5):494-503.

Levine, M., et al. 1999. Criteria and recommendations for vitamin C intake. *Journal of the American Medical Association* 281:1415-23.

Linderman, J., and K. Gosselink. 1994. The effects of sodium bicarbonate ingestion on exercise performance. *Sports Medicine* 18:75-80.

Linderman, J., L. Kirk, J. Musselman, B. Dolinar, and T. Fahey. 1992. The effects of sodium bicarbonate and pyridoxine-alpha-ketoglutarate on short-term maximal exercise capacity. *Journal of Sports Sciences* 10:243-53.

Linossier, M.T., D. Dormis, P. Bregere, A. Geyssant, and C. Denis. 1997. Effect of sodium citrate on performance and metabolism of human skeletal muscle during supramaximal cycling exercise. *European Journal of Applied Physiology* 76:48-54.

Lukaski, H., et al. 1996. Chromium supplementation and resistance training: Effects on body composition, strength, and trace element status of men. *American Journal of Clinical Nutrition* 63:954-65.

MacDougal, J.D., G.R. Ward, D.G. Sale, and J.R. Sutton. 1977. Biochemical adaptation of human skeletal muscle to heavy resistance training and immobilization. *Journal of Applied Physiology* 43:700-703.

MacDougall J.D. et al. 1995. The time course for elevated muscle protein synthesis following heavy resistance exercise. *Canadian Journal of Applied Physiology* 20:480-86.

Mahesh, V.B., and R.B. Greenblatt. 1962. The in vivo conversion of dehydroepiandrosterone to testosterone in the human. *Acta Endocrinologica* 41:400-406.

Maresh, C., C. Gabaree, J. Hoffman, D. Hannon, M. Deschenes, L. Armstrong, A. Abraham, F. Bailey, and W. Kraemer. 1991. Anaerobic power responses to amino acid nutritional supplementation. *International Journal of Sports Nutrition* 1:366-77.

Matson, L., and Z. Tran. 1993. Effects of sodium bicarbonate ingestion on anaerobic performance: A meta-analytic review. *International Journal of Sports Nutrition* 3:2-28.

McNaughton, L. 1992a. Bicarbonate ingestion: Effects of dosage on 60s cycle ergometry. *Journal of Sports Sciences* 10:415-23.

McNaughton, L. 1992b. Sodium bicarbonate ingestion and its effects on anaerobic exercise of various durations. *Journal of Sports Sciences* 10:425-35.

McNaughton, L.R. 1990. Sodium citrate and anaerobic performance: Implications of dosage. *European Journal of Applied Physiology* 61:392-97.

McNaughton, L., K. Backx, G. Palmer, and N. Strange. 1999. Effects of chronic bicarbonate ingestion on the performance of high-intensity work. *European Journal of Applied Physiology* 80:333-36.

McNaughton, L., and R. Cedaro. 1992. Sodium citrate ingestion and its effects on maximal anaerobic exercise of different durations. *European Journal of Applied Physiology* 64:36-41.

McNaughton, L., R. Curtin, G. Goodman, D. Perry, B. Turner, and C. Showell. 1991. Anaerobic work and power output during cycle ergometer exercise: Effects of bicarbonate loading. *Journal of Sports Sciences* 9:151-60.

McNaughton, L., S. Ford, and C. Newbold. 1997. Effect of sodium bicarbonate ingestion on high-intensity exercise in moderately trained women. *Journal of Strength and Conditioning Research* 11:98-102.

Mero, A. 1999. Leucine supplementation and intensive training. *Sports Medicine* 27:347-58.

Mero, A., et al. 1997. Effects of bovine colostrum supplementation on IGF-1, IGG and saliva IGA during training. *Journal of Applied Physiology* 83:1144-51.

Mero, A., H. Pitkanen, S.S. Oja et al. 1997. Leucine supplementation and serum amino acids, testosterone, cortisol and growth hormone in male power athletes during training. *Journal of Sports Medicine and Physical Fitness* 37:137-45.

Mitch, W.F., M. Walser, and D.G. Spair. 1981. Nitrogen sparing induced by leucine compared with that induced by its keto-analogue, A-Ketoisocaproic in fasting, obese man. *Journal of Clinical Investigation* 67:553-62.

Mitchell, J.B., P.C. DiLauro, F.X. Pizza, and D.L. Cavender. 1997. The effect of pre-exercise carbohydrate status on resistance exercise performance. *International Journal of Sport Nutrition* 7:185-96.

Mortimore, G.E., A.R. Poso, M. Kadowaki, and J.J. Wert. 1987. Multiphasic control of hepatic protein degradation by regulatory amino acids, general features and hormonal modulation. *Journal of Biological Chemistry* 262:16322-27.

Moukarzel, A.A., O. Goulet, J.S. Salas et al. 1994. Growth retardation in children receiving long-term parenteral nutrition: Effects of ornithine alpha-ketoglutarate. *American Journal of Clinical Nutrition* 60:408-13.

National Coffee Association, National Soft Drink Association, Tea Council of the U.S.A., and information provided by food, beverage, and pharmaceutical companies and J.J. Barone, H.R. Roberts. 1996. Caffeine Consumption. *Food Chemistry and Toxicology* 34:119-29. [Online]. Available: www.cspinet.org/new/cafchart.htm.

National Research Council. 1989. Recommended dietary allowances. National Academy Press, National Academy of Sciences.

Nissen, S., L. Panton, J. Fuller, D.Rice, M.Ray, and R. Sharp. 1997. Effects of feeding beta- hydroxy-beta- methylbutyrate (HMB) on body composition and strength of women. *Federation of American Societies for Experimental Biology Journal* 11:A150.

Nissen, S., L. Panton, R. Wilhelm, and J. Fuller. 1996. Effect of beta- hydroxy-beta-methylbutyrate (HMB) supplementation on strength and body composition of trained and untrained males undergoing intense resistance training. *Federation of American Societies for Experimental Biology Journal* 10(3):A287.

Nissen, S., R. Sharp, M. Ray, J. Rathmacker, D. Rice, J. Fuller, A.Connelly, and N. Abumrad. 1996. Effect of leucine metabolite beta- hydroxy-beta- methybutyrate on muscle metabolism during resistance-exercise training. *Journal of Applied Physiology* 81 (5):2095-2104.

Nissen, S., R.L. Sharp, L. Panton, M. Vukovich, S. Trappe, and J.C. Fuller. 2000. Beta-Hydroxy-Beta-Methylbutyrate (HMB) supplementation in humans is safe and may decrease cardiovascular risk factors. *Journal of Nutrition* 130:1937-45.

Noonan, D., K. Berg, R.W. Latin et al. 1998. Effects of varying dosages of oral creatine relative to fat free body mass on strength and body composition. *Journal of Strength and Conditioning Research* 12:104-8.

Pakkanen, R., and J. Aalto. 1997. Growth factors and antimicrobial factors of bovine colostrum. *International Dairy Journal* 7:285-97.

Panton, L.B., J. A. Rathmacher, S. Baier, and S. Nissen. 2000. Nutritional supplementation of the leucine metabolite beta-hydroxy-beta-methylbutyrate (HMB) during resistance training. *Nutrition* 16:734-39.

Parry-Billings, M., and D.P.M. MacLaren. 1986. The effect of sodium bicarbonate and sodium citrate ingestion on anaerobic power during intermittent exercise. *European Journal of Applied Physiology* 55:524-29.

Pauli, D.F., and C.J. Pepine. 2000. D-ribose as a supplement for cardiac energy metabolism. *Journal of Cardiovascular Pharmacology and Therapeutics* 5:249-58.

Pearson, D., Hamby, D., Russel, W., and Harris, T. 1999. Long-term effects of creatine monohydrate on strength and power. *Journal of Strength and Conditioning Research* 13 (3):187-92.

Peeters, B.M., C.D. Lantz, and J.L. Mayhew. 1999. Effect of oral creatine monohydrate and creatine phosphate supplementation on maximal strength indices, body composition, and blood pressure. *Journal of Strength and Conditioning Research* 13:3-9.

Pettegrew, J.W., J. Levine, and R.J. McClure. 2000. Acetyl-L-carnitine physical-chemical, metabolic, and therapeutic properties: Relevance for its mode of action in Alzheimer's disease and geriatric depression. *Molecular Psychiatry* 5:616-32.

Poortmans, J.R., and O. Dellalieux. 2000. Do regular high protein diets have potential health risks on kidney function in athletes? *International Journal of Sport Nutrition and Exercise Metabolism* 10:28-38.

Rasmussen, B.B., et al. 2000. An oral essential amino acid-carbohydrate supplement enhances muscle protein anabolism after resistance exercise. *Journal of Applied Physiology* 88:386-92.

Rawson, E.S., M.L. Wehnert, and P.M. Clarkson. 1999. Effects of 30 days of creatine ingestion in older men. *European Journal of Applied Physiology*. 80:139-144.

Rennie, M.J., and K.D. Tipton. 2000. Protein and amino acid metabolism during and after exercise and the effects of nutrition. *Annual Review of Nutrition* 20:457-83.

Rowbottom, D.G., D. Keast, and A.R. Morton. 1996. The emerging role of glutamine as an indicator of exercise stress and overtraining. *Sports Medicine* 21:80-97.

Sahlin, K., and A. Katz. 1993. Adenine nucleotide metabolism. In *Principles of Exercise Biochemistry*, edited by J.R. Poortmans, 137-53. 2d. ed. Vol. 38. Basel, Switzerland: Karger.

Saint-John, M., and L. McNaughton. 1986. Octocosanol ingestion and its effects on metabolic responses to submaximal cycle ergometry, reaction time and chest and grip strength. *International Clinical Nutrition Review* 6:81-87.

Salvioli, G., and M. Neri. 1994. L-acetylcarnitine treatment of mental decline in the elderly. *Drugs Under Experimental and Clinical Research* 20:169-76.

Sandstedt, S., L. Jorfeldt, and J. Larsson. 1992. Randomized, controlled study evaluating effects of branched chain amino acids and alpha-ketoisocaproate on protein metabolism after surgery. *British Journal of Surgery* 79:217-20.

Sapir, D.G., P.M. Stewart, M. Walser et al. 1983. Effects of alpha-ketoisocaproate and of leucine on nitrogen metabolism in postoperative patients. *Lancet* 1 (8332):1010-4.

Schena, F., F. Guerrini, P. Tregnaghi, and B. Kayser. 1992. Branched-chain amino acid supplementation during trekking at high altitude. The effects on loss of body mass, body composition, and muscle power. *European Journal of Applied Physiology* 65:394-8.

Smeets, R., et al. 2000. Oral supplementation with bovine colostrum (Intact) improves sprint performance in elite field hockey players. *Journal of Strength and Conditioning Research* 14:370.

Soderlund, K., P.D. Balsom, and B. Ekblom. 1994. Creatine supplementation and high-intensity exercise: Influence on performance and muscle metabolism. *Clinical Science* (Colch) 87:120-1.

Stout, J., J. Eckerson, D. Noonan, G. Moore and D. Cullen. 1999. Effects of 8 weeks of creatine supplementation on exercise performance and fat-free weight in football players during training. *Nutrition Research* 19 (2):217-25.

Tarnopolsky, M.A., et al. 1992. Evaluation of protein requirements for trained strength athletes. *Journal of Applied Physiology* 73:1986-95.

Tipton, K.D., et al. 1999. Post-exercise net protein synthesis in human muscle from orally administered amino acids. *American Journal of Physiology* 276:E628.

Tipton, K.D., and R.R. Wolfe. 2001. Exercise, protein metabolism, and muscle growth. *International Journal of Sport Nutrition and Exercise Metabolism* 11:109-32.

Tipton, K.D., et al. 2001. Timing of amino acid-carbohydrate ingestion alters anabolic response of muscle to resistance exercise. *American Journal of Physiology* 281:E197-206.

Tiryaki, G.R., and H.A. Atterbom. 1995. The effects of sodium bicarbonate and sodium citrate on 600 m running time of trained females. *The Journal of Sports Medicine and Physical Fitness* 35:194-8.

Uralets, V.P., and P.A. Gillette. 1999. Over the counter anabolic steroids 4-androsten-3,17-dione; 4-androsten-3B,17B-diol; and 19-nor-4-androsten-3,17-dione: Excretion studies in man. *Journal of Analytical Toxicology* 23 (5):357-66.

Vanakoski, J., V. Kosunen, E. Meririnne et al. 1998. Creatine and caffeine in anaerobic and aerobic exercise: Effects on physical performance and pharmacokinetic considerations. *International Journal of Clinical Pharmacology and Therapeutics* 36:258-62.

Vanbourdolle, M., L. Cynober, N. Lioret et al. 1987. Influence of enterally administered ornithine alpha-ketoglutarate on hormonal patterns in burn patients. *Burns Including Thermal Injury* 13:349-56.

Vandenberghe, K., M. Goris, P. Van Hecke, M. Van Leemputte, L. Vangerven, and P. Hespel. 1997. Long-term creatine intake is beneficial to muscle performance during resistance training. *Journal of Applied Physiology* 83 (6):2055-63.

Van Gammeren, D., D. Falk, and J. Antonio. 2001. The effects of supplementation with 19-Nor-4-androstene-3,17-dione and 19-Nor-4-androstene-3,17-diol on body composition and athletic performance in weight-trained male athletes. *European Journal of Applied Physiology* 84 (5):426-31.

Van Someren, K., K. Fulcher, J. McCarthy, J. Moore, G. Horgan, and R. Langford. 1998. An investigation into the effects of sodium citrate ingestion on high-intensity exercise performance. *International Journal of Sport Nutrition* 8:357-63.

Verbitsky, O., J. Mizrahi, M. Levin, and E. Isakov. 1997. Effect of ingested sodium bicarbonate on muscle force, fatigue, and recovery. *Journal of Applied Physiology* 83:333-37.

Volek, J., N. Duncan, S. Mazzetti, R. Staron, M. Putukian, A. Gomez, D. Pearson, W. Fink, and W. Kraemer. 1999. Performance and muscle fiber adaptations to creatine supplementation and heavy resistance training. *Medicine and Science in Sports and Exercise* 31 (1):1147-56.

Vukovich, M., R. Sharp, L. Kesl, D. Schaulis, and D.King. 1997. Effects of a low-dose amino acid supplement on adaptations to cycling training in untrained individuals. *International Journal of Sports Nutrition* 7:298-309.

Vukovich, M., N. Stubbs, R. Bohlken, M. Desch, J. Fuller, and J. Rathmacher. 1997. The effect of dietary beta- hydroxy-beta- methylbutyrate (HMB) on strength gains and body composition changes in older adults. *Federation of American Societies for Experimental Biology Journal* 11:A376.

Vukovich, M., N.B. Stubbs, and R.M. Bohlken. 2001. Body composition in 70-year-old adults responds to dietary beta-hydroxy-beta-methylbutyrate similarly to that of young adults. *Journal of Nutrition* 131 (7):2049-52.

Walker, L., et al. 1998. Chromium picolinate effects on body composition and muscular performance in wrestlers. *Medicine and Science in Sports and Exercise* 30:1730-6.

Wallace, M., et al. 1997. Effects of short-term creatine and sodium phosphate supplementation on body composition, performance and blood chemistry. *Coaching and Sport Science Journal* 2:30-34.

Wallace, M.B., et al. 1999. Effects of dehydroepiandrosterone vs androstenedione supplementation in men. *Medicine and Science in Sports and Exercise* 31:1788-92.

Webster, M., M. Webster, R. Crawford, and L. Gladden. 1993. Effect of sodium bicarbonate ingestion on exhaustive resistance exercise performance. *Medicine and Science in Sports and Exercise* 25:960-65.

Welbourne, T.C. 1995. Increased plasma bicarbonate and growth hormone after an oral glutamine load. *American Journal of Clinical Nutrition* 61:1058-61.

Wernerman, J., F. Hammarqvist, and E. Vinnars. 1990. Alpha-ketoglutarate and post-operative muscle catabolism. *Lancet* 335:701-3.

Williams, J.H., J.F. Signorile, W.S. Barnes, and T.W. Henrich. 1988. Caffeine, maximal power output and fatigue. *British Journal of Sports Medicine* 22:132-34.

Williams, M., R. Kreider, and D. Branch. 1999. *Creatine: The power supplement*, 15. Champaign, IL.: Human Kinetics.

Williams, M.H. 1998. *The ergogenics edge*, 249. Champaign, IL.: Human Kinetics.

Witter, J., P. Gallagher, D. Williamson, M. Godard, and S. Trappe. 2000. Effects of ribose supplementation on performance during repeated high-intensity cycle sprints. Paper presented at the Midwest Regional Chapter of the ACSM, October.

Wolfe, R.R. 2000. Protein supplements and exercise. *American Journal of Clinical Nutrition* 72 (2):551S-557S.

Wolinsky, I., ed. 1998. *Nutrition in exercise and sport*. Boca Raton, FL: CRC Press.

Yakolev, N.N. 1975. Biochemistry of sport in the Soviet Union: Beginning, development and present status. *Medicine and Science in Sports* 7:237-47.

Yen, S.S., A.J., Morales, and O. Khorran. 1995. Replacement of DHEA in aging men and women. Potential remedial effects. *Annals of the NY Academy of Sciences*. 29 (774):128-142.

Zaragoza, R., J. Renau-Piqueras, M. Portioles et al. 1987. Rats fed a prolonged high protein diet show an increase in nitrogen metabolism and liver megamitochondria. *Archives of Biochemistry and Biophysics* 258 (2):426-35.

Ziegenfuss, T.N., and D.J. Kerrigan. 1999. Safety and efficacy of prohormone administration in men. *Journal of Exercise Physiology*$_{online}$.

Ziegler, T.R., et al. 1990. Safety and metabolic effects of L-glutamine administration in humans. *Journal of Parenteral and Enteral Nutrition* 14:137S-146S.